Carrying to Term

If you're not sure where to start, download our free
list of lab work and forward by
Dr. Jordan Robertson ND at
miscarriagedownload.drjordannd.com

Copyright ©2018 Dr. Jordan Robertson, ND
Revised 2020.

All rights reserved. No part of this publication may be reproduced, stored in a retrieval system or transmitted in any form or by any means – electronic, mechanical, photocopying, and recording or otherwise – without the prior written permission of the author, except for brief passages quoted by a reviewer in a newspaper or magazine. To perform any of the above is an infringement of copyright law.

Book design by First Choice Books

10 9 8 7 6 5 4 3

Carrying to Term

A practical guide to reducing
your miscarriage risk.

Dr. Jordan Robertson, ND

To Parker and Charlie
xoxo

CONTENTS

Preface 1

Ch. 1 Recurrent Pregnancy Loss 5

Ch. 2 Risk Assessment 9

Ch. 3 Before You Are Tested 19

Ch. 4 The Diagnosis 40

Ch. 5 You Are What You Eat 103

Ch. 6 Stress And Exercise 116

Ch. 7 Nutritional Supplements 121

Ch. 8 You. Can. Do. This 155

Afterword 157

References 171

PREFACE

THE UNTHINKABLE

I understand.

I had trouble putting into words what I had lost, after my first miscarriage. I was only seven weeks pregnant — with a blighted ovum that had not developed past week three. Despite knowing I was pregnant for only two and a half weeks, I had somehow over the course of those sixteen days rewritten my future.

My life in those two weeks had zoomed into another land where I was a mom, and we were a family, and then zoomed back to where it was before. Did I have a terrible life before I got pregnant? "No". Did I even plan to get pregnant? "No". Was the timing even good for me to get pregnant? "No" (I was half way through my last year of Naturopathic Medical school). But in two weeks I had rewritten my future to include another person, and then I found out that this person didn't exist.

Some time after — who knows how long, the next few months were a blur, I found the words to describe the experience better, but still feared sharing them with people other than my husband.

I was mourning my future.

I wish I could say I only received the most encouraging and supportive advice, but many people struggle to find the right words of comfort in difficult times. Not realizing how painful it was, so many could only muster the phrase, "well it must not have been meant to be".

After braving my red eyes in public again, I was flooded with stories from friends and family members that had also miscarried. I was shocked. Why didn't I know there were so many sad stories lurking in our circle of friends and family? Why did all of these people keep their pain to themselves?

I experienced two more miscarriages that same year. The second was just before I wrote my naturopathic medical board exams, and the third occurred the week I got my results. Stress, was likely a contributing factor.

I needed a plan.

Diving into the literature to see what had been studied helped me to understand the cause of my miscarriages and to cope better with my loss. As a woman, and Naturopathic Doctor, I owe it to you to help you better understand this topic.

My goal with this book is to provide you with resources to help you understand not only the why, but also the things that may help you carry a pregnancy to term. Specifically, this book will provide you with information to ensure you ask the right questions, get a thorough assessment, learn

PREFACE

how to reduce your own risk, and who to approach for the next steps in your journey to stay pregnant.

Whether your wish is to have a natural birth, or improve the success of your IVF, you should finish this book with a resource list including; lab work you need to have done, dietary changes that every woman should make, and a list of supplements that may help, depending on your diagnosis. Each suggestion is geared to improve the likelihood of you carrying a pregnancy to term. By no means is this book an exhaustive resource, nor a replacement for a good quality practitioner experienced in treating miscarriage — but it should empower you and guide you through a self-advocacy process.

Let's get started.

CHAPTER 1

RECURRENT PREGNANCY LOSS

Some of the most exciting research I have done on miscarriage so far is about the assessment process of women who are at risk of, or who have already miscarried. Every country assesses women differently, and every medical governing body has weighed in on the topic. In my experience, this rarely trickles down to actual clinical practice and how women are assessed and treated in real life.

I think with all of the wonderful advancements we have seen in reproductive medicine; we have got a little lost along the way when it comes to assessment. Technology has played a vital role in carrying pregnancies to term. Quite literally almost every diagnosis of 'infertility' can result in a full-term pregnancy—with the right procedure, and the right amount of cash. This has downgraded the importance of finding out the actual reason behind your issues. Do we care if you have polycystic ovaries, premature menopause or uterine fibroids if the treatment options are the same? Do we need to test Vitamin D, for celiac disease, or progesterone deficiency if we give all of three women the same drugs during their IVF cycle?

If we look at assessment from a public health perspective, maybe we don't care to dig that deep. Perhaps we don't need to know what the underlying pathology or imbalance in one particular patient is when statistically we know that we can improve her chances of success by following the protocols written in stone.

> That's not good enough for me.

Why, because for each woman the results of her assessment matters, especially when the solutions to the problems are not hard to treat. The success of IVF cycles is low on the whole. Risk of miscarriage is high in women who have already had one or two. So, if simple tests and simple solutions can improve our odds, why don't we care?

If miscarriage is "so common", then when do we test you? Do we get bent out of shape after one? Or do we wait for the recommended 3-4 before we get curious about what's going on? Conventionally we wait until a woman satisfies the diagnosis of "recurrent pregnancy loss" before we start to look for the reason. I'll tell you, after 3-4 miscarriages, women have had just about enough trauma. Even without knowing the research, I think we can agree we should be asking questions sooner.

What does the research say? For many events that happen in medicine, the frequency that they occur changes the assessment, the investigation and the diagnosis. With miscarriage, we seem to have fallen into the one size fits all trap. Here's an example:

If you get a couple of hives once, we probably don't care. We also probably cannot figure out what caused it, nor do we try. We chalk it up to chance and don't think twice about it. If you get them again that same year, we'd probably say, "Hey, there are those hives again". We'd try and link the two events – but we probably can't, and still probably don't care.

Now, if you get hives every day for a year, two things happen. One, we care more. Two, the reason you're getting hives is not the same as your two random episodes the year before. Those two times were from strawberries (very allergic/histamine fruit by the way), and now instead of it being a simple oral allergy to a fruit you occasionally have, you have a systemic, or whole body, disease that causes hives. The reason changed. A systemic disease would not cause hives randomly twice a year, and we upped the ante on assessment because the stakes feel higher.

Now with miscarriage, we are finding the complete opposite. The reason you have your first miscarriage is the same reason you have your second, third or fourth[1,2]. So, I'll ask you, when do we test you?

The research has suggested that instead of waiting until women satisfy the diagnosis of recurrent pregnancy loss, we should check them sooner. They indicate after the second[2], but I recommend after your first. Better yet, let's think proactively. If you're reading this in the waiting room of a fertility clinic, I have news for you, you're at risk. To mitigate this risk, my recommendation would be that a miscarriage assessment is part of a preconception plan for all women—especially since most of these solutions are general health changes.

CHAPTER 2

RISK ASSESSMENT

So how do we know if you're at risk? I find it ironic that in our/my generation we spent our whole teenage years—and most of our twenties, trying our damnedest not to get pregnant. What we, failed to realize, is just how hard it was going to be to get pregnant when we were ready.

Infertility, in general, is on the rise, and miscarriage rates have likely climbed along with them. The reason for this in-tandem increase in infertility and pregnancy loss, is that many of the very conditions that cause infertility also cause miscarriage. Talk about a double whammy. You couldn't get pregnant, now you did, and now you're more likely to miscarry than other women.

In this section, I'm going to walk you through the underlying conditions that increase your risk of miscarriage. If you fall in any of these camps, (or what we commonly see is that women fall into more than one camp), then you will want to keep reading the next section where I talk about which lab tests I recommend. But first I want to start by articulating my position that miscarriage is a public health problem.

Specifically, miscarriage reflects the health of our generation of women, and how stress, hormones, and the environment are playing a role. Now if you know you're one of my Poly Cystic Ovarian Syndrome girls, don't skip ahead. As I said, you may fall into more than one camp, and many of the solutions are similar across the board.

POLY CYSTIC OVARIAN SYNDROME OR PCOS is a complex metabolic condition that causes multiple hormone imbalances. The root of these issues is altered insulin sensitivity and elevated androgens (testosterone and DHEA). These changes make it very difficult for women to manage their weight, causes hair loss on your head, hair growth everywhere else and significant cycle problems. Women with PCOS may never get a period, cycle irregularly (32-40+ day cycles) or bleed monthly. Either way, many cycles are likely "anovulatory", meaning that no egg is released because no egg can mature in this hormonal soup. Women with PCOS are at an increased risk of infertility, but when they finally do get pregnant, they are at an increased risk of miscarriage too.

The reason PCOS causes miscarriage is not what most people, or even most doctors would probably guess. Funnily enough, we can take an egg out of a woman with PCOS and donate it to another healthy woman with great success[3] and during controlled IVF cycles with 'excellent' embryos, women with PCOS still miscarry more[4]. What does that mean? The egg is not the problem. Women with PCOS are not at an increased risk of abnormal eggs. The eggs cannot get going. Even though testosterone is high, estrogen is high (and low at the same time), and progesterone is low if things do actually come together to fertilize the egg, it is an underlying problem with insulin and blood sugar that is the difference maker for miscarriage[5].

Women with PCOS are not necessarily overweight, but in all women, lean or heavy, issues with insulin release and sensitivity are a problem, and this appears to be the contributing factor to the increased risk of miscarriage. If women with PCOS are heavier than their ideal body weight they are at even higher risk, with some studies showing miscarriage after IVF being as high as 25% in overweight women (while only 11% in the average BMI group)[6].

LAB TESTS TO CONSIDER: *Day 21 hormones to detect ovulation, fasting insulin, fasting glucose, Vitamin D, homocysteine.*

LUTEAL PHASE DEFECT (LPD) has been the bane of my naturopathic diagnostic existence. It means something particular: your uterus is not as mature as it should be for the day of your cycle you are on. For example, your uterine lining may look like day 17, but you're on day 23. The problem with this is how the hell do we know what day your uterus thinks you're on? The short answer is we don't — unless we biopsy your uterine tissue. No woman is lining up for a biopsy to determine the maturity of her uterine lining, and we don't have the resources for it anyways.

Now here is the problem: lots of things will cause an "apparent" luteal phase defect. Specific elevations in hormones can prevent the lining from maturing, low hormones can prevent the lining from maturing, and so can a straight-up lack of ovulation—which could be from anorexia, low body weight, stress and a few other causes. Conventional medicine hates this. A kinda-diagnosis that could be caused by lots of underlying things that does not always show up on blood work. Perfect. Now, what do we do?

If you have the clinical signs of LPD, then you need a good work up with a curious practitioner. You should have your prolactin, cortisol, and body fat analysed to look for "secondary" causes. True LPD is likely caused by a normally ovulated egg, that doesn't produce enough progesterone to mature the uterus in time for its own arrival. See, after the egg is released, the collection of cells it leaves behind in the ovary (the corpus luteum) produces a lot of progesterone to mature the uterine lining rapidly. In women with LPD, we think the "CL" does not work well or is destroyed by oxidative stress (the opposite of anti-oxidants)[7]. Women with LPD also seem to require more progesterone for their uterine lining to mature. Your uterine cells are not as sensitive to progesterone, so you need higher levels to do the job. So, the gist is, you don't make progesterone, and you need more than other women. Yikes.

Clinically this immature uterine lining trickles down to spotting before your period, short cycles (<25 days), poor implantation and increased risk of miscarriage—or just not getting pregnant in the first place.

LAB TESTS TO CONSIDER: *Mid-Luteal (approximately day 21) progesterone or 3 consecutive days of progesterone readings, prolactin, androgens (testosterone, DHEA), cortisol.*

CHAPTER 2 — RISK ASSESSMENT

PREMATURE OVARIAN FAILURE (POF), or "early menopause" is a challenging diagnosis. In women destined for this diagnosis, their ovarian decline likely started as many as twelve years before things finally show up on lab work or before cycles begin to change[8]. These women are often in fertility clinics for hyper-stimulation protocols to try and recruit more eggs to be fertilized in vitro. Some women have POF from environmental exposures such as chemotherapy[9] and some women may be genetically wired to be at risk. Either way, if these women do get pregnant, we want to hang on to that egg for dear life.

Predicting the success of an IVF procedure in women with POF is difficult. In general, having an elevated FSH (Follicle Stimulating Hormone) even once in your life predicts a poorer success rate in POF[10], but the research also suggests that we should not discourage women under 35 from doing any procedure based on her lab work alone[11,12].

We have found in the literature that women diagnosed with POF may also have other underlying autoimmune issues, with the most relevant to miscarriage being autoimmune thyroiditis (Hashimoto's Thyroiditis)[13]. These women may also have altered white blood cell counts—possibly pointing to autoimmunity and low vitamin D.

LAB TESTS TO CONSIDER: *Complete blood count, Vitamin D, Day 3 FSH, AMH.*

HASHIMOTO'S THYROIDITIS (Autoimmune Thyroiditis) is a common cause of "low thyroid" that has a significant impact on fertility and carrying to term. Pregnancy is a stress on the thyroid, and even slightly low thyroid before conception can be a risk for early pregnancy loss[14]. Elevated antibodies against the thyroid are enough to diagnose the condition. We have one problem. Conventionally we never test antibodies in a walking-well woman without apparent signs of low thyroid. A large commission on thyroid and pregnancy in France has suggested that if we universally screen women for Hashimoto's when they consider getting pregnant, we will find double the thyroid disease[15]. Meaning we let a lot of women walk around with low-grade thyroid inflammation unchecked and untreated.

The challenge with Hashimoto's is that, unlike plain old hypothyroidism, our targets for thyroid function change. Meaning, if you have Hashimoto's, we need to medicate you until your thyroid works better than average. The target TSH for women with Hashimoto's should be below 2.5, and yet we often let women walk around with a TSH up to 4 or 5 before we consider offering support[14]. Why Hashimoto's causes miscarriage is a bit of a mystery. We also see elevated thyroid antibodies in women with celiac disease, and other high-miscarriage risk conditions, so apparently it is worth testing, and using thyroid hormone where appropriate to get these numbers in check.

LAB TESTS TO CONSIDER: *TSH, T4, T3, TPO, Anti-TG, Vitamin D*

CHAPTER 2 — RISK ASSESSMENT

HYPERHOMOCYSTEINEMIA (HHCY) is a bit of a go-between condition. As we understand it right now, Hhcy shows up in almost every other high-miscarriage risk condition, from PCOS to Anti-Phospholipid Syndrome (APS). It has made understanding Hhcy difficult because as of writing this book, we have no idea why it would show up in seemingly unrelated conditions. Homocysteine is an amino acid that technically should be turned into more healthy amino acids like cysteine. This process is dependent on folic acid, B12, B6 and a few other nutrients, which if we mess with either the intake (vegans), the absorption (celiac) or the use (genetic issues with folic acid that we will touch on later) we get a backlog of homocysteine instead. So, in part, homocysteine is a marker for something else going wrong further up the chain[16]. But aside from being a 'biomarker' of another problem, homocysteine alone causes issues with the development of the placenta, and by itself causes miscarriage. So regardless of the underlying cause, if a woman tests positive for Hhcy, we should be addressing it head-on[17].

LAB TESTS TO CONSIDER: *Homocysteine, B12, RBC folic acid, and screening for other related conditions such as celiac disease or PCOS.*

AUTOIMMUNE DISEASE (Celiac, Crohn's, Lupus, etc.) has been considered a risk factor for miscarriage for years. Each autoimmune condition increases the risk of miscarriage but also increases the chance that you will be diagnosed with another high-miscarriage risk condition. The nutritional demands or deficiencies that occur with autoimmune disease are likely a culprit, and in addition to managing the disease itself, women should be screened for common nutritional deficiencies that may worsen their chances of carrying to term.

LAB TESTS TO CONSIDER: *inflammatory markers, B12, ferritin, Vitamin D, homocysteine.*

ANTIPHOSPHOLIPID SYNDROME (APS) is mostly a clotting problem but shows up as a fertility problem because of the blood vessel development that occurs when the placenta begins to take shape. This condition results in slightly later miscarriages (week 8-9), and unfortunately one of the diagnostic criteria is 3-4 consecutive miscarriages. Women with APS also have elevated antibodies, and the higher the antibodies are, the worse their chances of carrying to term. APS also presents with elevated homocysteine much of the time and is treated with anticoagulants to help women carry to term.

LAB TESTS TO CONSIDER: *Anti-cardiolipin antibodies, anti-lupus antibodies, homocysteine, vitamin D*

HYPERPROLACTINEMIA is one of our luteal-phase-defect-like conditions that should be ruled out as a cause of miscarriage in all women with a previous miscarriage, or who have short cycles, spotting between periods or significant breast pain with their cycle. Prolactin is produced in the pituitary in the brain and is our lactation hormone. The problem is that it can be over-expressed under stress, or with an abnormal pituitary growth (prolactinoma) and can suppress parts of your cycle, damage your corpus luteum — say goodbye to progesterone production and increase miscarriage risk. There is a reference range, and if you are frankly out of range, you may require medication to lower it, as well as a MRI scan to ensure it is not from a growth on your pituitary.

LAB TESTS TO CONSIDER: *Prolactin measured in the morning, at least two hours after waking.*

ENDOMETRIOSIS should be on your list to exclude if you have significantly painful menstrual periods. It is an inflammatory condition where uterine tissue grows in the pelvis, outside the uterus, and creates significant inflammation and pain with your cycle, as well as between cycles. Women often have pain with intercourse, pain with bowel movement and every-day pain that usually requires medication to manage. The gold standard to rule-in this condition is a laparoscopic assessment, where they insert a camera through an incision into the pelvic cavity to look around, and the remove endometriosis lesions at the same time. So again, we are faced with the condition that can only be assessed through surgery, biopsy or looking inside. Sigh.

Endometriosis causes miscarriage for a million reasons. Inflammation, immune dysfunction, physical changes in the uterus all contribute to an increased miscarriage rate[18]. Women with endometriosis have lower success with IUI and IVF than women with almost any other cause of infertility. We have our work cut out for us.

Recently a blood test that was traditionally used to follow uterine or ovarian cancer patients was found to be elevated in most cases of endometriosis. CA-125 can be used to rule-in endometriosis with high accuracy, but if the test is negative, you may still have it as it is not accurate at ruling it out[19]. I usually suggest my women with chronic pelvic pain be screened for endometriosis with the blood tests, so we can be sure we are barking up the right tree.

LAB TESTS TO CONSIDER: *CA-125, Vitamin D.*

CHAPTER 3

BEFORE YOU ARE TESTED

Before you go and get tested, it's important that you do a bit of homework to better understand your own situation a bit better. What I mean by that is that you need to become in tune with your own health, and your own cycle in order to help us help you. If you are unsure how long your cycle is, whether or not you have cervical mucous, or when to have intercourse, it's time to get up close and personal with your own cycle and symptoms. It's the first step to figuring out what's going on.

Menstrual cycles can be broken down into a few phases, and being aware of what is going on in each phase can give us clues to why you may be at risk for miscarriage; if you are unfamiliar with your cycle, this where you should start. The first day of your period is the first day of full real flow. If you spot before your period, you need to track this; it might be a sign of low progesterone, which is a risk factor for miscarriage. During your cycle and leading up to ovulation, we consider this the follicular phase. This is where the follicle grows to get ready for release and ovulation. We can test certain hormones in this phase to check how responsive your ovaries are, which we discuss in the next section. After ovulation is the luteal phase, and from the perspective of miscarriage, this is often where we focus most of our efforts. During the luteal phase hormones are high, and the uterus matures and prepares for implantation.

What I would suggest is to start tracking your cycle in detail. Track the number of days it is, when you experience changes to cervical mucous, and what your PMS experience is like. Whether you use paper and pen or an app, be sure to log all of these parts of your cycle. As a side note, I often use validated questionnaires in my practice to measure PMS symptoms in women. I prefer the Daily Record of Severity of Problems checklist, which you can find for free online. This checklist allows you to track your symptoms across your cycle, to see when they happen, and when things feel better or more severe. It's the gold standard for actually assessing PMS. Have a look, sometimes women are shocked that we would consider many of their symptoms part of a PMS experience.

WHAT TO TRACK TO ACCURATELY ASSESS YOUR OWN CYCLE

* **THE TOTAL LENGTH OF YOUR CYCLE.** This is first day of bleeding to the next first day of bleeding.
* **TOTAL NUMBER OF DAYS OF BLEEDING.** Include how heavy your period is. We usually ask women how often they have to change their protection as our gage.

- **WHETHER OR NOT YOU HAVE SPOTTING BEFORE YOUR FIRST REAL DAY OF BLEEDING.** Spotting can be a sign of low progesterone towards the tail end of your cycle. Brown or very minimal blood would be considered spotting.
- **CERVICAL MUCOUS CHANGES.** We expect this to occur half way through your cycle. Cervical mucous changes to a thicker egg-white consistency around ovulation.
- **YOUR PMS SYMPTOMS.** Include physical signs such as breast tenderness, bloating and headaches. Track your mood as well.
- **TRACK YOUR CRAMPS.** Include the number of analgesic pills you take monthly to control your symptoms.

PMS symptoms are not truly related to miscarriage, however they may point towards what your other challenges with fertility and miscarriage may be. PMS truly doesn't happen unless you ovulate. If you have some months that are easy breezy, and some months where you feel like Mrs. Jekyl and Mrs Hyde, then you may not be ovulating every month. Track your PMS to help us figure this out.

LABORATORY TESTING

Assessment for your miscarriage risk needs to be done carefully, and with a practitioner who is well versed in miscarriage and how to treat it. Conventionally we don't do a great job looking at "wellness" based assessment. Modern medicine is great at life and death (if I have appendicitis, I know where to turn), but not a great job with the subtleties of chronic symptoms or disease. I have been working on women's hormonal health my entire career, and never have I heard a conventional medical practitioner give a resounding "YES!" to testing hormones or even to testing nutrients related to hormones. We use the "she's not broke enough to hospitalize her, we don't need to fix it (her)" approach to women's health, and this pat-on-the-head tactic does one of two things: leaves women feeling disempowered about their health, or sends them to an off the grid practitioner, like me.

The rest of this section is a list of lab tests that you may want to consider if you have had a previous miscarriage, or if we think you're at risk. Not every lab needs to be done for every woman. I always tell my female patients, "lab work needs to tell us something we don't already know or change your treatment."

What I mean by this is that if we were going to do vaginal progesterone no matter what your lab work said, then don't do the labs. Or if we can tell by your clinical history that you bleed out a monsoon of blood every month, then maybe we don't need to test your iron to at least get you started on some iron supplements. Follow?

So, here's my advice: don't march into your doctor's office with the entire list.

Pick out the tests that you think are the most relevant to your case and ask for those. If they say no, reference my quote: "would it help us understand something we don't already know, or change my treatment?" or something like that. Medically their minds work the same as mine, the goals are just a little different. I want you never to miscarry again.

FEMALE HORMONE TESTING *(Day 3 FSH, Estradiol, Day 21 Serum Progesterone, Estradiol, FSH):* Relevant to PCOS, LPD and to assesses for premature ovarian failure.

Two kinds of scenarios land across my table when it comes to hormone testing. Women who have never had any done, and women who have had the wrong ones done. Never has a woman brought me the right lab work.

Testing your female hormones takes a bit of detective work. There are hormones made in your brain, which I refer to as your upstairs hormones, and there are hormones made in your ovaries: your downstairs hormones. You need both sets tested, and you need them done at certain times of the month. Testing progesterone and nothing else never teaches us where the kink in the chain is. We need to be specific in order to diagnose you accurately and treat you effectively.

FOLLICULAR PHASE HORMONES *(Day 3 FSH, Estradiol)*

Hormone testing is challenging because your hormone levels are different every single day of your cycle. When we test matters. Which means if you have been tested but did not go on a particular day, the tests were done wrong. The beginning of your cycle is when your brain is trying to recruit follicles to grow. FSH (follicle stimulating hormone) is released in a 'just right' amount to make this happen. If your FSH levels are high, it means your ovaries are not responding. We can use this number to predict your future likelihood of getting pregnant.

Elevated FSH (above 15-20 IU/L) is the first point of diagnosis for premature ovarian failure. Entirely outside the scope of this book to address this topic adequately, but POF is a significant cause of infertility in women and starts to show up years before you hit early menopause. We even think that women who are going to be diagnosed with POF may have reduced fertility for 8-10 years before we diagnose them[8]. Not great news.

If FSH is elevated even once, it means your likelihood of success is lower. If you are younger than 35, we should not use it to discourage you from doing any other fertility treatments[10], but if you are over 35, it requires a real serious conversation about how far and long you want your fertility treatments to go. Women with POF are at an increased risk of miscarriage, but maybe only if they are over 40. In a couple of studies, they did not see a huge correlation between recurrent pregnancy loss and POF in women under 40, but there seemed to be a connection in slightly older women[11].

We think the increased risk of miscarriage in POF is due to a "two-hit" hypothesis. Genetics may have created an accelerated ovarian age, versus your real age, and then if we throw any other single, even small risk on top of that, you are more likely to miscarry[13]. So, women with POF probably need to be more careful about their diet, environmental exposures and their nutrient intakes to prevent miscarriage than women without, but full disclosure—we don't know why you miscarry more, or indeed how to treat it. I don't discuss premature ovarian failure as its own chapter because the research is so weak. There's some information in the hormones chapter on the use of DHEA.

LUTEAL PHASE HORMONES *(Day 21 Progesterone, Estrogen, free Testosterone, FSH, LH)*

Testing in your luteal phase really should focus on determining if you ovulated and if you did not, where the kink in the chain is. Only testing your 'downstairs' hormones does not tell us what's wrong. If they are low, we don't know why. We have to test the 'upstairs' hormones to follow the path. Low progesterone in your luteal phase means you did not ovulate. You will find out later when I discuss treatment that yes progesterone supplementation is helpful, but no it does not make you ovulate.

This book is focusing on how to keep you knocked up. Which means I'm assuming a few things. Girl ovulates, boy meets girl (meaning sperm and egg), and we want to stay knocked up. Luteal phase defect (LPD) women ovulate but still have lower levels of progesterone than we need. If you have a single reading below 30 nmol/L (10 ng/mL) or three subsequent days in your luteal phase that total less than 93 nmol/L (or 30 ng/mL), then you likely have LPD, and you are at an increased risk of miscarriage. If your progesterone is 2 nmol/L (<1 ng/mL), then you did not ovulate at all, and you need another book. You probably still need this one, but you need to focus on ovulating first.

There's some fresh research on estrogen to progesterone ratios and PMS, but again, unrelated to miscarriage. The reason I test estrogen at all in the luteal phase is to look at whether a woman's cycle is suppressed centrally (upstairs/brain), peripherally (downstairs/ovaries). If you have had luteal phase timed blood work done, and your practitioner did not test your FSH you should have them all rechecked to really understand what's going on.

I wish I had more exciting things to say about progesterone testing. Unfortunately we don't really see a big connection between your actual progesterone levels and the likelihood of miscarriage. Meaning that we can't run the test, and then predict who will miscarry. We wish we could do that—it would make our lives so much easier.

We know that progesterone sensitivity is a problem, meaning that in many cases a woman's uterus is less responsive to this hormone than it should be, and we also know that treating women with progesterone—we will get to that later, helps women carry to term. But the real usage of a progesterone test at this point is to clarify whether or not women have ovulated. Ideally preformed around 7 days after ovulation (or around day 21) progesterone levels above 10 nmol/L (3.1 ng/mL) are indicative of ovulation. We usually like to see numbers higher than that, with numbers closer to 30 nmol/L (9.4 ng/mL) mid-luteal being ideal.

Your hormones need to be tested in your blood. I repeat. Your hormones need to be tested in your blood. I repeat. Your hormones need to be tested in your blood. Over the years, fancy tests involving saliva and urine have crept into the functional medicine scene, and make promises of better understanding your case, by looking at your special individual hormone magic, and then personalizing your treatment plan off of these special tests. I have a huge problem with expensive tests that don't tell us anything more than a cheap blood test, and urine and saliva progesterone levels don't tell us anything more than blood. Urine is a good surrogate measure for ovulation and costs way more than blood. Saliva isn't a great correlate for ovulation, because the reference ranges are kind of meaningless. All of the research on miscarriage has looked at serum progesterone. Not a single scrap of evidence has looked at the other methods of assessing progesterone or any of your other hormones for that matter.

Free Testosterone is the best measure for androgens in women with PCOS, and these levels are related to miscarriage rates[20]. If you want to be completely thorough, you can test total testosterone and SHBG too[21], but a free testosterone is the most reliable marker when it comes to PCOS and miscarriage.

VITAMIN D: Relevant to PCOS, POF, LPD, Hashimoto's Thyroiditis, Autoimmunity and nearly every other cause of miscarriage out there.

You're going to get the hint pretty soon that vitamin D is a big deal. It's involved in hundreds of hormonal and immunological processes and shows up in nearly every cause of infertility and miscarriage. Now, there is some question about how or why vitamin D is low in almost every woman who has miscarried and has created a bit of a chicken-and-the-egg scenario for researchers. Vitamin D is made when we are outside. What do we do outside? We exercise. So, is it a coincidence that vitamin D is low in almost every metabolic disease associated with obesity? Not really. Is it a coincidence that it is low in nearly every woman diagnosed with breast cancer—when being overweight is one of the most significant risk factors for breast cancer? Not really.

So, sceptics of the vitamin industry have claimed that vitamin D is just a surrogate marker for outdoor exercise. And they might be right. That said, when we watch women with infertility in studies, if we improve their vitamin D status they ovulate more, get pregnant more and miscarry less. Even if they sit inside on their ass. We should just be testing and treating women who are planning to get pregnant.

When I graduated from school, our 'acceptable' vitamin D limit was 40 points lower than it is now. We have changed our minds in the last ten years about how important it is, and what 'low vitamin D' really means. I would shoot for a value of over 110 nmol/L on your lab work. This number comes from a study where over 95 decreased risk of miscarriage, and over 112 increased live birth rates 4 fold[22].

CHAPTER 3 — BEFORE YOU ARE TESTED

FASTING INSULIN AND FASTING GLUCOSE:
Relevant to PCOS, LPD

> "I'm going to bet my chickens that you haven't had your fasting insulin tested. Ever."
>
> "Oh, yes I have!" (says every patient)
>
> **Proceeds to dig through purse/phone/tablet to find lab work from her latest physical**
>
> "A-Ha! Here it is"
>
> **Points to GLUCOSE (FASTING)**
>
> (Jordan does a face-palm for the third time that day)

Every woman who has had a physical exam done in her lifetime has had her fasting glucose tested. What were they looking for in a healthy young woman like yourself? Diabetes. Fasting glucose is a screening tool for diabetes. Public health screens patients every year, as it also only costs a couple of bucks, and when their blood sugar gets too high, we congratulate them and tell them they have diabetes.

The problem with fertility and miscarriage is that very few of you has diabetes. Fasting insulin on the other hand, rises YEARS — maybe even DECADES — before glucose ever rises, because fasting insulin is a measure of how well your body is coping with your weight, diet and carbohydrates, and often you can compensate quite well for years before you develop diabetes.

Fasting insulin is the culprit for the increase in miscarriage we see in PCOS. Funnily if we donate a PCOS woman's eggs to a woman who does not have PCOS, she does not miscarry as often[3] It is not the egg - it is the environment the egg is in. Elevated insulin means your body is leaning towards storage, growth and is struggling to manage your dietary carbohydrates (we will get to this later).

My goal for women is for their insulin to be in the bottom 25% of the reference range, and their HOMA-IR (a calculation that compares insulin and glucose) to be below 1.0. The fasting insulin range is looking for things other than what we are focused on such as insulin-producing tumors, and we want to tighten things up a bit to get the best outcome. Bottom quarter. In Canada, that's below 50 pmol/L on the chart.

THYROID FUNCTION TESTS *(TSH, T4/T3, TPO, Anti-TG):* Relevant to Hashimoto's Thyroiditis, Antiphospholipid syndrome, Women with a previously diagnosed celiac disease.

If you want to watch a Naturopath and a Medical Doctor fight, give them some lab work with a TSH of 3.5. I have had the good fortune of working with the family medical resident teams at my local hospital on integrative care options, and the only thing we fight about is TSH.

Fertility is a fantastic example of how thyroid function is supposed to go, and how we should be valuing it more in the general population. Always remember: we need your body to be functioning correctly to get pregnant. If you keep this in mind, the rest becomes easy. Sort of.

The most important part of this topic to remember is that TSH alone is not a helpful marker when it comes to miscarriage. TSH is a brain-based (or more accurately, pituitary based) hormone, that signals for your thyroid to produce more thyroid hormone. In hypothyroidism, when your thyroid is functioning sub-par, this number goes up as your brain sends a stronger signal to recruit your thyroid to work harder. When it comes to miscarriage, this number alone doesn't tell the whole story, but it's often the only number tested as part of regular physical exams or prenatal screening.

The reason TSH alone is not enough, is that the thyroid-driven cause of miscarriage actually stems from a condition called Autoimmune Thyroiditis, or Hashimoto's Thyroid, and in many of these women, their TSH never rises enough to get flagged that there's a problem. If women have antibodies against their thyroid, they have difficulty getting pregnant without medication, but if we never test the antibodies we never know if they are there.

So the short version is that you need a full thyroid panel including thyroid antibodies to assess miscarriage risk. The long and complicated answer to treatment is in the Hashimoto's chapter.

CA-125: Relevant to endometriosis

If you have struggled through your life with severe menstrual cramps, there's a chance that you may have endometriosis as part of your picture. Endometriosis is a strange bird, in that uterine tissue grows outside the uterus, and your immune system cannot take care of it. It leads to perpetual inflammation and increased local hormones. Up until recently, we could only confirm if women had endometriosis with laparoscopic surgery and scoping her abdominal cavity. The recent findings that the cancer antigen CA-125 may also be elevated in endometriosis has given us a non-invasive way of ruling in the disease[23,24]. Unfortunately, at this time a negative test does not rule it out - you could still have endometriosis and not have CA-125, but if the test is positive, it is almost a guarantee that you have endometriotic lesions, which will increase your miscarriage risk.

CORTISOL: Relevant to all women

Cortisol is our stress hormone that is released by our adrenal glands after a signal from our brain. Although not always well correlated to a woman's perception and experience of stress, if cortisol is elevated, it indicates an increased risk of miscarriage. Some studies have even shown that if your stress hormone goes up from conception to implantation, you're at an increased risk of miscarriage[25]. The utility of the test is helpful in women with 'unexplained miscarriage' or who identify stress as being a detriment to her health. I mentioned before that my three miscarriages were during the most stressful times of my life. Bang – bang – bang. I lost three babies in Naturopathic Medical school. I did not measure my cortisol until much later in life and then it was normal. I wish I had measurements when it mattered.

PROLACTIN: Relevant to LPD, shortened menstrual cycle (<25 days), women with significant breast pain during their period.

Prolactin is our milk-producing hormone, and I'm sure you have seen, heard, or experienced, breastfeeding lowers fertility and ovulation rates—although it is not your most accurate birth control so watch out! Prolactin causes a luteal phase-defect issue because it suppresses follicle development and ovulation, resulting in an incomplete cycle. Women with high prolactin will also have low progesterone, not because the prolactin lowers it, but because a cycle without an egg does not make any. It is important to distinguish between low progesterone as a result of high prolactin or actual LPD because the treatment is different. In true LPD we are looking at progesterone. With elevated prolactin, we need to calm that puppy down first, which may require a drug – unfortunately.

HOMOCYSTEINE: Relevant to PCOS, Antiphospholipid syndrome, Celiac Disease, Vegans and Vegetarians, women with a previous baby with neural tube defect, Down's syndrome or congenital/developmental abnormality, women with a prior pregnancy with pre-eclampsia, or other prenatal complications.

Homocysteine is a blood test, and because it is so important I wrote a whole bloody chapter about it. Homocysteine is a biomarker of nutritional deficiency, a flag for genetic issues and a signal for how much weight and obesity is playing a role in your miscarriage risk. The test is done fasted, or after a methionine load, which is an amino acid that gets turned into homocysteine. Most of the fertility research is on fasting homocysteine. Start there.

AUTO-ANTIBODIES: Relevant to women at risk for APS, with a family history of celiac, lupus, or who have already tested positive for Hashimoto's.

The curious thing about autoimmune disease, is that once it shows up in one spot in a patient, it's likely to show up in another spot. Women who test positive for Hashimoto's, celiac or lupus are at risk of miscarriage, and at risk of having other autoimmune diseases too. Your particular autoimmune condition may not be directly associated with miscarriage — such as Rheumatoid Arthritis, but it may not be your only autoimmune condition. I'm not suggesting that you go on a wild goose chase to find more problems, but I'm suggesting that you and your fertility team need to get really interested in your total health and narrow down if any other parts of your health should be screened. My suggestions specific to miscarriage is to test ANA (Lupus antibody), Celiac and Hashimoto's (TPO) as a start. If any of them are positive, regroup and talk to your practitioner about whether or not you should do more.

ALL THE OTHER TESTS: Relevant to every woman

Of course, we cannot possibly cover every single cause of miscarriage out there, and some are much better managed conventionally than the more hormone-related causes I have listed above. It is thought about a quarter of miscarriage are related to endocrine/hormone issues (PCOS, LPD, diabetes, thyroid, prolactin). I have included a few other causes above that appear to be on the rise in this generation of moms. The list below should also be considered as part of a complete workup:

* Uterine ultrasound to look at the structure, previous scars (Asherman's syndrome) or fibroids.
* Sexually Transmitted Disease screen to test for Chlamydia or Syphilis, which may cause chronic endometritis.
* Illicit drug use such as cocaine increases miscarriage risk
* Chromosomal abnormalities and advanced maternal or paternal age
* Workplace toxins (although none have been correctly identified, there's some evidence that hair stylists and shift workers may have more miscarriages than other professions).

OTHER TESTS THAT ARE NOT ASSOCIATED WITH MISCARRIAGE RISK—*but would be a good idea to do anyway.*

Now, this could be a long list. There are many tests we can do to understand your total health better. And since we already shook on it that your overall health impacts your fertility, I'm sure we agree (since you said you did!) that if there are parts of your health that are not well, then it is not helping our end game.

That all said, I'm cautious with how I present this list. I do thousands of medical tests at my office every year. But all of them have been medically necessary. Remember that "telling us something new, changing your treatment" always needs to apply. Doing tests because they are new, or cool is not good enough for me.

So! How do we marry the goal of understanding your total health and only doing tests that are medically necessary? It's a tough job. Usually, when I'm working with women, I present their tests in "need to know" and "nice to know" lists and "what else do we need to consider if we are still staring at each other in three months". This strategy seems to help us prioritize, plan and then have a contingency plan too.

If you were going to start a laundry list of other tests you should maybe have done, these are a few I would consider:

ADRENAL ANDROGEN TESTING (DHEA)

Androgens are quite involved in the pathogenesis of PCOS and can be the cause of some of the physical symptoms we see associated with it such as acne and hair growth. DHEA hasn't been found to be that helpful in the diagnosis or management of PCOS above a free testosterone level. I mentioned this earlier in the hormone section, but for completeness—if you are having your hormones tested—a DHEA value can be helpful to your practitioner.

B12

B12 levels on their own don't have tremendous relevance to miscarriage, but if chronically low, may point to another diagnosis such as celiac disease and if they are deficient, they may contribute to elevated homocysteine levels—which can be seen in strict vegetarians or vegans who don't supplement. Ideally levels should be comfortably above 200 pmol/L.

FERRITIN

Ferritin is a marker of iron storage in the body. It is more sensitive than Hemoglobin to tell us how sufficient your iron levels are and can easily fly under the radar as low, since so many women walk around tired anyway. Ferritin alone is not related to miscarriage, but this number will dictate whether a prenatal vitamin alone is enough to keep your iron levels high enough in pregnancy. If your ferritin is below 40 ug/L you should maybe talk to a practitioner about supplementing. The reference range lets us tired women walk around with levels as low as 5. Not a fantastic idea if you ask me. The other reason to test is how bloody long it takes for iron levels to be raised. It can take months of supplementation before ferritin begins to climb. If you have struggled with heavy periods, short cycles or spotting between periods this test should be on your hit list.

TESTS YOU DO NOT NEED

Why focus on this? Well, I have a couple of reasons. One is that some of these tests require medical visits, wait times for testing, scans and interpretation of your scans, and then follow up visits to go over the results. In other words: TIME.

If we make you wait a few months while we test you, and the results don't help us, all we have done is lost a few months.

The best example of this is a pelvic ultrasound for polycystic ovaries (PCOS). As you have read so far, PCOS is mostly a metabolic problem that ends up as a fertility problem. In some women, it causes multiple 'arrested' or immature follicles to collect in the ovaries, and these show up as cysts on ultrasound. So, doing an ultrasound could be a good idea, as it's still technically part of the diagnostic work up for PCOS. However, as far as screening for fertility and miscarriage, an ultrasound is useless.

A significant standards of care document on fertility looked at this very issue. Ultrasound results do not predict if you will miscarry[26]. Even if you have miscarried before. It does not predict your future chance of success. So, don't go. Or at least don't wait around for your results.

The other imaging that has no value is a uterine MRI. Previously recommended as part of a very comprehensive workup for women who may have anatomical problems with their uterus that are getting in the way of getting pregnant. Turns out waiting for a scan and waiting for the results don't get you any further ahead. Skip it.

The other reason that we would kibosh a particular test is if the solution for your condition will be the same, regardless of your test results. The best example of this is genetic testing or testing for MTHFR gene mutations. MTHFR is the folic acid-activation-pathway that we discuss in other sections. Some women struggle to make good-quality methylfolate from dietary or supplemented folic acid, putting them at risk of deficiency, neural tube defects and miscarriage. There is some growing body of evidence that these ladies may actually be worse off if we supplement them with plain old folate (as in most prenatal multivitamins) but as it stands right now, testing for MTHFR does not get you any further ahead than using methylfolate right out of the gates or using high dose 'normal' folate. I know I have colleagues that disagree with this statement, and perhaps even have helped some women get pregnant after testing for gene mutations. I'm just telling you the evidence. Right now, I don't think it is necessary[26].

Most other genetic tests are also not necessary, neither is testing an early miscarried embryo. If you have had late, and recurrent second or third-trimester miscarriage, it's another story.

The likelihood that you have made it to your adult life with a debilitating genetic defect that is also getting in the way of your fertility (such as Turner's syndrome) is low. However, talking with an experienced practitioner about your entire reproductive life such as when you had menarche, secondary sex characteristic development, and your body stature, may shed light on the necessity of this. Right now, as far as screening goes, it should not be anywhere near the top of the list.

CHAPTER 4
THE DIAGNOSIS

I have tried my best to cover almost every cause of miscarriage that we can assess and even threw in a chapter for you 'unexplained' women at the end. I had inherent difficulties breaking this all down into digestible sections for one reason.

Every single diagnosis we discuss increases your chance of having the other diagnoses, and every positive lab test you have increases your chance of having other positive lab tests.

What the hell do I mean by that?

It means that every cause of miscarriage is linked to every other cause of miscarriage. It says that every lab test is related to every other lab test. How we break this apart for some women is arbitrary. They are a "miscarrier" and should be treated as entirely and comprehensively as possible.

My focus of this book was is to give you enough tools to be adequately assessed in the first place. I want you to have some language to walk into your doctor's office with — rather than feeling unheard and confused. I have worked hard to create connections here that might be a light-bulb moment for you. I have worked hard to present what we know. But unfortunately, there's a lot we don't know.

Given that you bought a book on the topic, I likely don't need to convince you that your total health is related to your fertility. Try your hardest not to get hung up on fitting into any of these diagnoses 'boxes', like I said, falling in any box means you might belong in other boxes. Read all the sections through, get confident in how to approach this, and who to work with.

PCOS

If I had to choose one condition that was a good reflection of the state of our world and health as women, I'd select PCOS. It is a combination of our genetics, epigenetics (genetic changes over a short period like from mother to daughter, or in a single woman's lifetime), environment, diet, lifestyle, and stress. It is what's happening to women because of how we live, and how our lives are changing due to modern life. It is a topic for another time given how massive and complicated it is, and I know you're reading this to have fewer miscarriages, not to hear my version of what is wrong with the health of our women in general.

The reason I mention this, is to show you that not only is this as complex as all hell but also, that the solution has to be equally as complex and detailed, — not hard, just complex, to account for all of the facets of this condition.

There's just no way that putting women with PCOS under a standard IVF protocol will work as well as it could as if we addressed all of the ways her body is out of sync. Yes, we can force you to ovulate, yes, we can push the egg and sperm to meet up, but we cannot force you to carry to term. That is why you are reading this book in the first place.

We have had a hard time studying women with PCOS because, shockingly, you are not all the same. Some women have elevated levels of insulin, some have high testosterone, some are overweight, and some are lean. Some women get androgen symptoms (acne, hair growth) some don't. Most don't ovulate, and you all have trouble with fertility, so we usually pool you all together and study you together. Of course, there are problems with this, but we also haven't figured out a better way to do it. Sigh.

The next section will go through all of the symptoms of PCOS and will help you understand how to get properly assessed—but before we go there, I want to give you some insight on the condition in general.

What is happening in PCOS, whether you're overweight or not—is dysfunction in insulin and blood sugar regulation. This cascades all the way down to the level of the ovary, causing significant hormone disruption and stunted growth of your follicles. The eggs have a hell of a time trying to mature with such mixed signals, and as a result, many of them get partially developed, and often show up as cysts on ultrasound. Funnily, even if we don't see cysts, you can still have polycystic ovarian syndrome. I'm in favor of a name change.

CHAPTER 4 — THE DIAGNOSIS

The purpose of insulin in a healthy woman is to take carbohydrates from diet and deliver them to cells for use in energy production. Insulin puts fuel away into cells. In women with PCOS, not only do they make too much insulin (more storage of glucose than we want), their cells are not very responsive to it either. Even muscle cells have an altered response to insulin in women with PCOS. This is a whole-body situation but ends up creating a lot of problems with fertility.

Elevated levels of insulin change the kinds of hormones that are produced around the ovary. Usually a beautifully timed event, ovulation requires certain hormones to be released at certain times to have the egg grow and be released. High insulin causes a lot of testosterone to be created at the level of the ovary, and low levels of Estrogen. The complete opposite of what we need for proper egg development. These hormonal problems cause the follicles to 'arrest' in their development, and without an ovulated egg, there will be no progesterone production. I will address each lab test in the next section, but I'm starting with this conceptual idea of insulin first to show you that diet, is the first place to start. Yes, fertility treatments can fix the Estrogen and progesterone. But remember that they are the last step of a 1000 step process. I cannot tell you how many times I have seen women with PCOS get prescribed progesterone to fix their progesterone deficiency. Guess why it is low? Insulin. Starting at the top is how we fix the miscarriage issue.

The changes that occur in PCOS are similar to what we see in patients with diabetes and cardiovascular disease.

As a result, these women have inflammation in the blood vessels similar to what we would expect in an overweight diabetic male. Carrying to term requires you to produce new blood vessels in the placenta, and to create a healthy maternal-fetal bond that can nourish your baby and prevent miscarriage. In women with PCOS, their placenta essentially has cardiovascular disease as it is forming. The vessels are not as healthy as women without PCOS, and as a result, the maternal-fetal bond is impaired, which is likely a big trigger for the increase in miscarriage. In one study, they found that the worse a woman's androgens and insulin were, the fewer blood vessels she formed in her placenta[27]. I feel like that statement bears repeating: you cannot even make placental blood vessels if your insulin and testosterone are high.

No one has done the kind of research I want to see on PCOS and miscarriage. We have studies that show us that if women eat high fiber melba toast instead of regular melba toast that they have more regular menstrual cycles[28]. They are both terrible choices. Why they haven't studied complete diet overhauls with carbohydrate reduction, intermittent fasting and supplementation for reducing insulin release are beyond me. I already know that if you have read this far, you are way beyond the melba toast women. You want real change.

DIAGNOSING PCOS

The diagnosis of PCOS requires a bit of detective work because, like I mentioned, you are all different. Each and every lab test could be positive or negative in women with POCS. Drat. We hate when this happens in medicine. We want there to be a really solid line between having something and not. Wishy-washy is not medicine's forte because how on earth can we prescribe our set-in-stone treatment plan if we are not sure if you fit in the box (note the sarcasm).

Remember this before you start reading: having only a few of these symptoms may be enough to warrant investigation. Many women with PCOS continue to have regular cycles. They bleed, but it does not mean that they ovulate. These women often go un-assessed until they have tried to get pregnant for over a year.

SYMPTOMS OF PCOS

* Increased appetite or thirst
* Fatigue, especially after eating
* Difficulty losing weight
* Irregular or absent menses

PHYSICAL SIGNS OF PCOS

* Increased waist to hip ratio or abdominal weight carrying.

* The darkened skin under the armpits (*acanthosis nigrans*)
* Acne
* Male-pattern hair thinning or loss
* Increased unwanted hair growth (chin, upper lip, nipple)
* Increased body hair growth

LABORATORY MARKERS AND IMAGING TO DIAGNOSE PCOS

* Pelvic ultrasound is showing 'pearl strand' ovaries or multiple cysts on the ovaries.
* Elevated fasting insulin and glucose, or an oral glucose tolerance test.
* LH to FSH ratio greater than 2. **Note that women with PCOS may show a 'positive' result on home ovulation predictor kits every time they test because of chronically elevated LH levels**
* Elevated total and free testosterone and DHEA (androgens)
* Low Sex Hormone Binding Globulin (SHBG)
* Sex hormones to be completed around day 21 of the cycle to assess for ovulation.

ADDITIONAL LAB TESTS TO ASSESS MISCARRIAGE RISK IN PCOS

* Homocysteine
* Vitamin D

TREATMENT CONSIDERATIONS

Okay girl, here is the thing: this is going to be a bit difficult. Treating your PCOS is hard, complicated, and the results will not happen overnight.

> Sounds terrible, doesn't it?

Let me offer my two cents. It is only terrible because of the way we have created thoughts and expectations about medicine and health. When you are sick, we give you stuff, and right away, you get better. When you have a complex metabolic disease, we try to do the same thing. Treat you and make you better right away. This creates a couple of problems. First, it absolves us from being partially responsible for our health because we have made the solution about giving you stuff, and not making you change your habits. So, any time we make patients change instead of taking something, they find it hard and annoying. That takes-stuff-get-better-quick mentality has also given us expectations that are not realistic. We want to lose 40 lbs. right away — even though it took us YEARS to gain it. We want acne to vanish after avoiding dairy for one day — when the lesions have likely been brewing for weeks. Working on your PCOS is no different. It will take meals and meals to lose weight, days of exercise to lower your insulin, and months of supplementation to ovulate on your own.

So here is the silver lining. Most studies on reducing miscarriages are less than three months long. So, even though I'm advocating for long-term, sustainable changes to your diet, lifestyle and supplements, we can likely improve your chances of carrying to term in three months. You have to promise me though, that you won't abandon the plan once you have your first ultrasound. All of the things that make you miscarry when you have PCOS also make you a high-risk pregnancy. You cannot abandon the plan. Pinkie swear.

SUPPLEMENT TREATMENT OPTIONS FOR PCOS

* Vitamin D based on blood work to achieve sufficient levels
* Berberine 500 mg three times per day unless you are being treated with Metformin.
* Homocysteine lowering strategies: See Homocysteine chapter)
* Progesterone suppositories from day 14 to 28 each cycle, or after any fertility treatment such as IUI or IVF, and continued after a positive pregnancy test to week 9-12 gestation.

The supplements that have been studied explicitly for PCOS both correct the insulin/androgen problems and override the endometrial and blood vessel development issues that plague women with PCOS. Berberine is a blood-sugar lowering herb that acts very similarly to Metformin (I discuss this further in the next section). Berberine lowers insulin and has been compared head to head against Metformin to show even better live birth rates and reduced miscarriages[29]. Lowering homocysteine can be achieved through diet and a good quality multivitamin. I discuss this further in chapter eight.

Vitamin D and progesterone both improve uterine blood flow, uterine lining and may help women carry to term by supporting that maternal-fetal connection[22,30]. The only side effect of progesterone that has been noted is that its use may be correlated with having larger babies[31]. Overweight women with PCOS are also at risk of larger babies, so we may want to decrease the number of weeks you are exposed to progesterone, but this has yet to be well studied.

DIET RECOMMENDATIONS FOR PCOS

There are two sides of the diet story with PCOS: weight loss and low carb. Interestingly, either diet, without the other (weight loss with high carb[32] or low carb[33] with no weight loss) improves hormone levels and fertility. No study has tried both. Additionally, to date, no one has investigated the subject of diet and miscarriage. Those studies that have included diet have been underwhelming with regards to evidence and recommendations. For example, they may tell women to eat low carb, but then don't teach them to eat fruits and vegetables and nuts and healthy oils, all of which improve hormone levels in PCOS.

The weight loss part of the diet is essential. Even women without PCOS who are overweight are at an increased risk of miscarriage[6]. Technically women with and without PCOS who have a high BMI have the same level of risk. Weight loss is hard and slow. But even a modest reduction of 5-10 lbs. seems to improve hormone levels enough to lower risk of miscarriage, regardless of your starting weight. There are a million strategies for success with weight loss, and most of them are behavioral. For example, if you write down what you eat, and don't be too hard on yourself, you are more likely to achieve your goals.

Despite me wanting to see research on radical diets in PCOS, clinically the best diet we can pick for you, is the one you can do consistently for 3-6 months. So, if you cannot live a day without cheese then let's rework the rest of your diet to be low carb, geared for weight loss, with a side of cheese. Remember that I need you to do this plan for six months. Don't set yourself up for failure by adopting a hard-core plan. It's better to implement changes you can stick to over the long-term.

In general, when it comes to miscarriage, choosing lower glycemic index foods and higher fiber foods while increasing fat and protein, you will be on the right track. When done for six months in combination with other treatments (such as Metformin) a low GI diet reduces miscarriage in women with PCOS. In one study the addition of a low-GI diet to the rest of their fertility plan reduced miscarriage rates in women with PCOS to match the miscarriage rates of women without PCOS (meaning they got WAY better)[34].

If you want to get specific about it, about 40% of your calories should come from carbs (30% fat, 30% protein) and you should have a calorie deficit of 300-400 calories per day from your resting metabolic rate. You can use simple free apps or tracking software to plug in your data. Your diet really should be tailored to your needs, labs, goals etc. But generally speaking, if we move women closer to a 40% carb diet their hormones work better. Homocysteine, also goes up with increasing BMI and waist circumference, and so in addition to the supplements, adjusting your diet can improve that particular miscarriage-risk factor too. All the more reason to eat better.

OTHER CONSIDERATIONS

As I mentioned earlier, the type of research I would hope to see on PCOS has not yet been done. I like to focus on research that gives real, meaningful results, but when we are missing what we need, we might have to use sub-optimal studies to make decisions. As I have mentioned earlier, fertility research uses a lot of surrogate markers to track success. They look at blood levels of nutrients and hormones, without looking at the actual number of babies born. We want babies!

That said, there is one nutrient that I use routinely use for PCOS that has only been studied looking at surrogate markers for miscarriage. In this case, I don't care if it has not been studied, and I'm going to contradict my earlier rant about surrogate markers completely.

INOSITOL, which is a B-Vitamin-like, carbohydrate-like compound has been studied to death on the metabolic issues in PCOS. It lowers androgens, insulin[35] and even homocysteine[36]. It helps with weight management, reduces the risk of gestational diabetes[37] and is seemingly a prominent genetic-metabolic missing link in women with PCOS. But, we don't have a study looking at its use for miscarriage. Crap! So, this is one of those times that I would advocate for treating the whole-picture/problem, rather than having a narrow laser focus on just reducing miscarriage. Inositol makes women with PCOS better. Let's use it, and maybe the research will catch up to us one day. I am only addressing this nutrient here, and not in the treatment chapters, because it only applies to PCOS, and as I said, it is a whole-body approach to treating women with this specific diagnosis. The trick with inositol is to get the right dose. 4 grams per day, (or 2 grams divided morning and night) is the dose that has the most favorable data for lowering androgens, insulin and homocysteine. There are a lot of negative studies that use 1-2 grams total. I cannot tell if it is a dose-response relationship, but positive studies use 4 grams, negative ones use 1-2. Let's agree to use 4.

MEDICATIONS THAT LOWER MISCARRIAGE

Given that insulin and blood sugar are the root issues in women with PCOS, it is not surprising that we have toyed with diabetic medications to try and fix it all. Metformin is the drug-of-choice when it comes to PCOS, and the benefits seem to extend beyond insulin and glucose.

Metformin improves the hormone environment around the ovary and encourages lower androgens, and better ovulation rates. It also enhances luteal phase progesterone, likely by enhancing ovulation[26,38]. Up until 2012, we did not think Metformin had any effect on miscarriage. It seemed to get women pregnant but did not help them stay pregnant. Some interesting data came out in the last few years that might explain why.

Metformin seems to work better if you're halfway to getting better without it. *Say what?* What I mean is, if your hormones are not entirely out of whack and if you are not as obese or overweight as you could be, Metformin will prevent miscarriage[39]. It is our ladies who have the greatest imbalances that it might not be effective. Enter the interdisciplinary approach!

The research done since 2012 have pointed out that if we combine treatments focusing on a diet with Metformin, we can lower miscarriage rates. Especially if the two are done together over a period of six months[39].

Metformin does not come without side effects, with the majority of them affecting the digestive system. A probiotic may reduce the side effects you experience, but so might a lower dose. I have seen many different prescribing practices with Metformin over the years. Some women do better on a sustained release capsule; some do better with three doses per day. You may have to play around with it a little — with your doctor — to avoid having diarrhea and an upset stomach. Berberine has been studied head to head against Metformin with equally as good results for miscarriage, and fewer side effects[29]. The challenge is the lack of safety data in pregnancy for Berberine. We know without a shadow of a doubt that Metformin is safe in pregnancy, we cannot be quite as confident with berberine. My take is, if you literally cannot tolerate the Metformin, then Berberine is a better option. If you can tolerate it, stick with the drug, and of course do the diet.

We haven't studied any other drugs in women with PCOS to assist with their fertility. Yes, there are other drugs, and yes, they lower insulin and sugar, but we don't know if they help with fertility. There are also drugs that treat the androgen symptoms of PCOS such as spironolactone, but the majority of these drugs are contraindicated in pregnancy, so maybe best left for a time when you're done having kids.

A SIDE NOTE ON BIRTH CONTROL PILLS

If you have had PCOS with irregular cycles, you have likely been prescribed an oral contraceptive at some point in time. There's a bit of a myth that you need to 'detox' from being on any contraceptive drug before you try and get pregnant — this is not true, especially for women with PCOS.

Oral contraceptives lower your testosterone and it takes a few months after stopping the pill for those androgen levels to go back up. That means that your first few months after stopping the pill might be your best chance of ovulating on your own and carrying to term. No detox necessary.

LUTEAL PHASE DEFECT

The term Luteal Phase Defect will likely in the next ten years undergo some diagnostic evolution, much like PCOS did ten years ago. We used to think PCOS was just "cysts on the ovaries" until we figured out it was a complex diabetes-like metabolic disorder, and cysts did not even need to be there for there to be a problem.

Right now, LPD is referring to the maturation of your uterus in the second two weeks of your cycle after ovulation. To have an LPD means that your uterus did not prepare for implantation, and when the egg makes it there, it is not ready to be a great host. The timing of uterine maturation is complicated, with hormonal cues making changes to blood vessels and the immune system to get ready to grab hold of, and then develop a placenta, with that egg.

So where is the problem? The problem is that about ten different conditions can cause uterine-maturation-timing issues, and have been collected together, and casually called LPD. In medicine, we hate this. We hate when multiple underlying causes produce the same diagnosis. When things like this happen, we also start to consider the syndrome itself a myth, and there are multiple papers and position statements that say that LPD is not a real thing[40].

CAUSES OF A LUTEAL PHASE DEFECT

* No ovulation, so no progesterone is produced in the luteal phase
* Inadequate production of progesterone from the corpus luteum (the part of the follicle left behind after ovulation).
* A uterus that is not receptive to progesterone, even if enough is present.

I'm sure you can see the need for some improvement on the definition of LPD. We cannot call infertility from someone who is underweight the same as infertility from someone who has high levels of prolactin, the milk-producing hormone. It just does not work for our linear-fit-in-this-box medical system. But for now, I'm going to lump all you lovely ladies into the same box. The end-stage problem is the same, and your lab work from the previous chapters will help sort out what the underlying issues are. You still have an LPD, so read on sister.

DIAGNOSING LPD

I'm sure after reading you're starting to suspect that you might be one of my LPD ladies. Which, but the way does not exclude you from one of the other possible diagnoses either. Lucky you! Two high-risk camps. Check the symptoms below to find out if LPD may be the cause of your miscarriages, and if you have got some previous blood work at home, you can check it against these lab tests I recommend.

PHYSICAL SIGNS

- A cycle that lasts less than 21 days total
- A cycle that lasts longer than 40 days total
- Spotting before the first real day of your period
- Low body weight, a BMI of less than 18, or low body fat %
- Significant breast pain each month, or leakage from your breasts

LABORATORY MARKERS & IMAGING

- Uterine biopsy in the luteal phase showing poor maturation (totally not a practical test, but technically this is the gold standard for diagnosis)
- Three consecutive days of progesterone readings (I suggest day 19-22) with the total of these three readings less than 93 nmol/L (30 ng/mL).
- A single progesterone reading in the mid-luteal phase less than 12 nmol/L (3.7 ng/mL)
- Elevated cortisol levels
- Elevated prolactin (PRL) hormone

* High androgens (testosterone, free androgen index, DHEA)

OTHER SIGNALS TO CONSIDER LPD AS A DIAGNOSIS

* High-intensity exercise 3-5 days per week
* Signs of an elevated stress response

TREATMENT CONSIDERATIONS

The treatment strategies for LPD need to extend beyond the risk of miscarriage because we think some of the underlying causes are related to 'oxidative stress' and poor ovulation. Both of these things are full body issues and slapping some progesterone on the problem may not be enough to solve it.

As I noted earlier in this chapter, LPD can be caused by multiple hormone imbalances, and the treatments to consider will depend on which hormones are out of whack. If prolactin is high, you need to consider Chaste Tree (Vitex) as a treatment[41,42]. If your cortisol is off, then we should be addressing stress and the adrenal glands. If you're getting on the right track with your hormones, we should see changes in your cycle length, less spotting and less PMS symptoms such as breast tenderness.

Regardless of the underlying "cause" of your LPD, all women that we suspect have luteal phase hormonal problems benefit from antioxidant support. Mistimed uterine maturation and poor progesterone production occur in all cases, with all LPD women producing less progesterone than they should. Interestingly the uterus is also not as responsive to progesterone even if levels are within range in women with LPD. You don't produce enough, and if you do, your uterus does not respond that well[7].

Oxidative stress is the exact opposite of antioxidants, which is a term thrown around to describe many natural health products. There are natural oxidative and anti-oxidative processes happening in your body all the time, and in a healthy body, with a healthy diet, we can counteract the oxidative stress easily. Exposure to the environment, an unhealthy diet or other physiological stressors—such as the inflammation from an autoimmune disease, increase the amount of oxidation, and it may start to outweigh the number of antioxidants in the system. Leading to inflammation which wreaks havoc on healthy bodily processes.

Women with LPD have been shown to have higher markers of oxidative stress in their bodies than women without, and if we look at your lifestyles, you all tend to participate in more activities that are known to increase oxidative stress such as smoking. You personally may not, but as a group, women with LPD smoke more, are more overweight and have more autoimmune disease. Whether LPD women are genetically wired to need more antioxidants or whether they do things that lower their antioxidants—such as smoking—is still up for debate, but interestingly the treatment focus is around improving antioxidant levels.

SUPPLEMENT TREATMENT OPTIONS FOR LPD

* Vitamin C 750 mg per day as a supplement (not through food)[43]
* Melatonin 3 mg at bedtime each night[44,45].

So, in all likelihood, there are WAY more antioxidants than the two listed above that would help with luteal phase defect. But, I promised earlier only to show you the things that had clinical evidence. Interestingly, there are thousands of articles looking at antioxidant support for farm animals. No joke. We know that changes to daylight and antioxidant status have a significant impact on an animal's fertility, but we haven't spent time looking at how that impacts the farmer? Honestly, science is so confusing sometimes.

Vitamin C is likely the most well-known antioxidant, even though it is not the 'strongest'. If you think that "Vitamin C enriched" OJ is a good source, think again. The 100% daily value listed on your foods and juices are 100% at a very low level. About 100 mg. Vitamin C recommended daily intakes were developed based on the amount you need to not be at risk for scurvy. "Optimal health" is not a consideration for most recommended daily intakes. Let me be the first to tell you if you are anywhere close to getting scurvy, you are also not getting pregnant. It does not take much Vitamin C as a supplement to have a positive impact on your fertility. The studies that have used Vitamin C for LPD used only 750 mg[43]. When dosed to women with LPD for just a month, Vitamin C improved progesterone levels and pregnancy rates (although not miscarriage rates). I know we are talking about miscarriage but getting to the root of the issue is essential. Reducing oxidative stress is good. Vitamin C is cheap. Just take it.

Melatonin is prescribed primarily for sleep, but it is first and foremost an antioxidant. Melatonin has been studied as a way to protect eggs that are being used for IVF because uniquely to other forms of fertility support, the eggs in IVF get exposed to the outside air! Melatonin, when given to the egg donor/mom-to-be, reduces the oxidative stress that the egg endures when exposed to the ambient air in the fertility clinic[46,47]. *Cool eh!* Melatonin, given even for a short duration, protects the ovary from oxidative stress and increases its ability to produce progesterone after ovulation. I would recommend that you take it nightly throughout your cycle. Melatonin also supports a better stress response and can influence cortisol levels in a positive way.

DIET RECOMMENDATIONS FOR LPD

The diet recommendations for LPD are not that different than what we usually suggest for women with low fertility. Urban-woman lousy behavior increases your risk, so look at that section and be sure that caffeine, alcohol, smoking, high saturated fat, sugar, and low nutrient foods are starting to exit your life. We want healthy oils (olive, avocado, nut) and nutrient-rich foods—bring on the fruits and veggies! We also know that women with LPD often under-eat.

So, from a dietary perspective, you likely have some room to grow!

Multiple sources can help you figure out what your caloric requirements are. Whether or not you need to lose weight, you cannot eat much less than a 300-calorie deficit from your basic-needs before you start to create some alarm bells in your body. Crash dieting is a thing of your past. Our bodies are wired for famine, and if you show it famine, you will shut down reproduction. We don't make babies if there is not enough food to go around. Makes sense does not it? So, start by figuring out what your needs are, and whether or not you need to lose weight. Track your diet for a week using a free diet tracker and figure out if your calories are hitting your needs. Most women in my practice under-eat some of the time, which either leads to overeating at other times or just a general state of under-nutrition. Your foundational health needs to be taken care of to carry to term.

OTHER CONSIDERATIONS

The other considerations for LPD mostly come from the multiple cause of this mistimed uterine prep and should be individualized based on what you and your practitioner find from your blood work. The herb I would be most likely to look at in women with short cycles, and high-normal prolactin would be Chaste Tree. This herb is one of my favorites, as it is hormone-regulating, PMS-busting abilities are unmet by any other treatment we have (conventional or integrative). It constitutes 30% of the prescriptions for PMS in Germany by Medical Doctors, whereas 30% of our North American women get an antidepressant[48]. Chaste Tree can lower prolactin and improve cycle length in women with short cycles and has been compared head to head with drug therapy with pretty good results. Unfortunately, we don't have research on Chaste for fertility per se, which is why it is mostly a side-bar recommendation for women with LPD. It is working on underlying processes, but it might not reduce your risk of miscarriage directly.

If your androgens are elevated (testosterone and DHEA) you may also struggle with LPD-like symptoms, and your treatment plan should include ways of lowering these hormones. Weight loss and nutrients like two heaping tablespoons of ground flax, inositol and resveratrol, the grape-antioxidant, all lower androgens and may support your underlying issues.

The other considerations for LPD are to find the areas of your health that are seemingly unrelated to your miscarriages and get them under control. I have advocated throughout the entire book that women with recurrent miscarriages need a competent, experienced practitioner. I will repeat it! You need a competent, qualified practitioner.

MEDICATIONS THAT LOWER MISCARRIAGE

Low progesterone is likely the last step of a thousand step process in LPD. However, when it comes to preventing miscarriage, slapping a band-aid on the problem long enough for the placenta to start making progesterone on its own seems to work[49]. Progesterone is safe and should be used liberally in women we think are at risk for low progesterone or miscarriage. I have never ever uttered the phrase, *"shoot, I wish we hadn't used progesterone"*, but have met hundreds of women that wished they had. The risks are low, and the benefits are high. Most fertility clinics are willing to prescribe suppositories for you to start the day after your procedure, until you have an established pregnancy. If you are trying to get pregnant naturally, there is evidence that we might want to use progesterone every month until you get pregnant in the luteal phase of your cycle[50]. Yes, this is a heavy-handed approach. Talk to your practitioner about their comfort prescribing this. The progesterone needs to be done vaginally, so prepare yourself with some panty liners! It can be a messy treatment. Topical (on your skin) and oral progesterone are not as effective when compared with vaginal[7].

PROGESTERONE RECOMMENDATIONS FOR LUTEAL PHASE DEFECT

* Progesterone suppositories from day 14 to 28 each cycle, or after any fertility treatment such as IUI or IVF.

I have left out discussing the other drug options for LPD, mostly because there aren't any. LPD is often managed in a fertility clinic, and whether you get clomiphene, IVF or other interventions, you should be appropriately supported with progesterone.

If your prolactin is very mildly elevated, I would not suggest using a drug to lower it. Bromocriptine is the most commonly prescribed dopamine agonist that lowers prolactin, and although there is no evidence that it causes any congenital disabilities, we have insufficient evidence that it helps reduce miscarriage—and one study that showed an increase in miscarriage[51]. Bromocriptine has some evidence for improving luteal phase symptoms associated with LPD such as a short cycle or breast pain. Chaste Tree may be just as effective if you're a high-normal prolactin lady anyways. In my opinion, stick with the herb. If your prolactin is elevated, you really should be evaluated for a prolactinoma (a tumor that makes prolactin) with an MRI of the brain. If you have a tumor that produces prolactin, you likely need drug therapy to manage it, but you should do a lot of other miscarriage prevention at the same time.

ENDOMETRIOSIS

Endometriosis has been a bit of a pet project of mine since I was a third-year undergraduate student. At that time, I wrote a paper on the newly discovered immune dysfunction in women suffering from this condition. My paper discussed that endometriosis has an auto-immune-like tendency and a cancer-like tendency at the same time. I chose to do the paper after coming across the diagnostic criteria for the condition and wondering if I had struggled with it myself.

The goings-on of endometriosis include uterine tissue growing outside the uterus. We don't know how it gets there — although we have always assumed that it backs up the fallopian tube (retrograde menstruation aka backwards blood flow), but we don't have a way of explaining how some endometriosis can show up in other weird spots, like the lungs. Either way, not only does the uterine tissue end up somewhere it is not supposed to, it continues to respond to your cycle. As your hormones fluctuate, the tissue grows and bleeds — with nowhere for the blood to go.

Enter: crazy pain and inflammation.

Now if your immune system was well and good, it would have no problem cleaning up stray cells that had found themselves somewhere they were not supposed to be. We know this because almost every woman has backwards menstruation every once and a while. But not every woman ends up with satellite lesions growing in her abdomen. So, on the cancer-like side of things, endometriosis evades detection and being cleaned up by your immune system. On the auto-immune side, the immune cells that are hanging around in your abdomen seem to perpetuate the situation rather than fix it. Everyone is having a party in your abdomen but for all the wrong reasons.

Women with endometriosis experience often profound menstrual cramps or even pain all month long, and struggle with getting pregnant in the first place. They struggle to get pregnant naturally, and they also have lower IVF success than other women[18,52]. This indicates that just by manipulating the hormones and forcing the situation, we are still missing the big picture of this condition. The immune system.

So, what does this have to do with miscarriage? Well as we have seen in other chapters, the immune system has a significant role to play in whether or not you carry to term. Chronic inflammation anywhere in the body seems to put us at risk for poor implantation or recurrent pregnancy loss, and in endometriosis, the inflammation is right in the front row—your uterus.

Unfortunately, we haven't studied endometriosis and miscarriage much, so my thoughts on the subject are much broader than in women with other causes of their miscarriages. The take-home message is that we cannot slap one magic-bullet solution on women with endometriosis. You all need less inflammation, less pain and a more effective immune system. How? Keep reading.

DIAGNOSING ENDOMETRIOSIS

Up until recently, the only way to rule-out endometriosis was to have laparoscopic surgery. They surgically go in with a camera and often remove the lesions they discover, all at the same time. It is still the gold standard, and even CT and MRI are not doing as good a job of identifying endometriosis as well as having a surgeon go in and look.

If the only way to assess women is through surgery, we likely have always underestimated how many women in the population have it. We cannot just grab 1000 women and send a camera inside to see the actual percentages in the population can we? If you have stepped up your medication to manage your cramps because Advil and Tylenol no longer cut it, have pain during bowel movements or sex—or some of the other symptoms listed below, then maybe you should be assessed a little closer.

Over the last few years, we have seen some research on a cancer marker called CA-125, which has been found to be a relatively accurate way of ruling-in endometriosis[19,23,24]. CA-125 is present in gynecological cancers, but also in endometriosis—and testing positive almost guarantees that you have endometriosis. Unfortunately, just because you test negative does not rule it out (false negatives are known to happen) but it is a reasonable place to start given that the other diagnostic option is going under the knife. It is also not that expensive of a test. Win-win.

SYMPTOMS OF ENDOMETRIOSIS

* Severe menstrual cramps
* Cramps and pelvic pain at other times of the month not associated with your period.
* Pain during intercourse or bowel movements.

LABORATORY MARKERS AND IMAGING

* Previous or current endometriosis lesions discovered or removed on laparoscopy. Even if this was found in

your teen years and treated, the chance of recurrence is very high.
* Suspected endometriosis lesions on CT or MRI
* Elevated CA-125

ADDITIONAL LAB TESTS TO ASSESS MISCARRIAGE RISK IN ENDOMETRIOSIS
* Vitamin D
* Ferritin and other markers of iron deficiency from heavy menstrual periods

TREATMENT CONSIDERATIONS

As I mentioned in the last section, endometriosis is a complex condition, with inflammation, hormones and the immune system interacting in a bit of a messy situation. We have been studying the *why* of endometriosis for years. Trying our damnedest to figure out why this happens in some women, and not others. What we haven't spent a lot of time on, is researching miscarriage in women with endometriosis.

In general, the treatment considerations for endometriosis should focus on lowering inflammation and improving antioxidant capacity. Although we haven't spent time studying it concerning pregnancy, pelvic pain and pain medication use decrease in women with endo if we improve her intake of antioxidants and supplement her with antioxidants. Even if you are going to do some significant drug therapy before your IVF cycle, we know we can improve the quality of life of you women just by having your nutritional intake and supplement intake focused on antioxidants. I usually suggest to my endo women that they track their analgesic use each month. We should see a reduction in the amount and the strength of pain meds required to manage your condition. Even downgrading from opioids to Advil is a win. Track it, and you should see some shifting with what I recommend here for miscarriage.

Some of you have actual physical issues as a result of this disease. Fibroid-like lesions, adhesions, scar tissue, or actual endometriosis lesions on your ovary ('chocolate cyst') all get in the way of getting pregnant. Especially fibroids and uterine scar tissue—these are the most linked with actual miscarriage. If you have been recommended for surgery, it might be the best way to go. Unless surgery damages your actual ovary[53], surgery seems to improve fertility in women with endometriosis.

SUPPLEMENT TREATMENT OPTIONS FOR ENDOMETRIOSIS

* Vitamin C 1000 mg and Vitamin E 1200 IU daily for antioxidant support[54]
* Melatonin 3-10 mg nightly for antioxidant and pain support[55]
* Omega-3 fats from fish oil to reduce inflammation[56]
* Vitamin D tested and treated to correct the deficiency[57,58]

One of the significant challenges in treating women with endometriosis is that the vast majority of conventional treatment options impair your fertility, and you have to come off them to even try to get pregnant. So, integrative supports not only have to help your chances of staying pregnant, but they also have to reduce your pain and inflammation, because you have discontinued the drugs that were helping you manage your symptoms.

Antioxidants are essential in the reduction of inflammation and can also help decrease the need for pain medication throughout the month when you discontinue your birth control or take out your IUD to prepare for fertility. Vitamin C has been well studied orally, and we have some emerging animal data that even vitamin C injections may help reduce the burden of disease[59]. I cannot wait for this to be studied in humans. Like the LPD section, we have reviewed Vitamin C and E, but in all likelihood, other antioxidants are beneficial, we have just considered the most popular ones first. Cheap and easy, Vitamin C and E are an excellent place to start.

Melatonin is an essential supplement for women with endometriosis. Interestingly, we know that women who work shift (and are awake when they are supposed to be sleeping) have lower levels of melatonin and increased risk of endometriosis and that women with confirmed endometriosis have lower levels of melatonin in their uterus than women without. Strange but true connection. Melatonin's most significant role in the body is as an antioxidant and is highly related to fertility in animals. It is likely because as the days get longer or shorter, there are more or fewer resources to go around for baby animals. It is a cool evolutionary thing that animals do naturally. Don't make a baby if resources are going to be scarce in 6, 9, or however many months it takes them to grow a baby.

There are a few cases of really high dose melatonin — combined with progesterone—suppressing ovulation in women. Low dose is fine, 3-10 mg, when taken nightly, improves pelvic pain in women with endometriosis and contributes to a less inflamed, more anti-oxidative environment in the uterus. Less pain for the women studied meant they reduced their opioid intake and took less pain medication overall. While you prep for your fertility care this sounds like a great idea.

Not surprisingly, based on what you are about to read in the diet section, fish oil and omega-3s have a positive impact on endometriosis. Women with the disease not only eat less fish but have a distorted ratio between omega-3s and more inflammatory fats such as Arachidonic Acid (AA). This imbalance means that when your uterine lining sheds, it is set up for more pain and inflammation from the get-go. Supplementing back in omega-3s is a good idea, as is eating more fish.

Vitamin D has been a suspect in the pathogenesis of endometriosis, given its concentration in the uterus, and it is immune-regulating properties. We haven't yet seen a cure-effect with giving vitamin D supplements, but we still don't want any of our fertility patients to walk around deficient. Test and treat. If you're deficient, you need it. If not? Congratulations! You must get more sun than the rest of us! Remember that Vitamin D is a prescription in some jurisdictions, and you may need to ask your practitioner if you need more than an over the counter dose.

DIET RECOMMENDATIONS FOR ENDOMETRIOSIS

* Reduce saturated fat from animal products and meat
* Increase fruit and vegetable intake
* Increase omega-3 fat intake from fish
* Include soy protein regularly in the diet
* Decrease alcohol intake

I have been following the research on diet and endometriosis for 15 years. Initially, what sparked my interest, was the apparent environmental influence of xeno-estrogens (chemical estrogens) on monkey models of endometriosis[60]. This research is old but keeps rearing its head to try and explain why some women struggle and some don't. There is a particular industrial compound group called dioxins that are endemically in our food supply and environment. They are in everyone's life, whether we like it or not.

Rhesus monkeys are a great animal model for endometriosis. Some unlucky female monkeys have endometriosis naturally, and we found by observing them, that the more dioxin exposure they had in their lifetime, the more likely they were to develop the disease—and the more severe their disease was.

It is always hard to prove causation in humans. It took us years to 'prove' smoking caused cancer. So we cannot conclusively say that dioxins cause endometriosis. That said, we know that women with endometriosis have more dioxins in their pelvic cavity than women without, detoxify it slower than women without, and may eat more of it through higher meat diets than women without[61]. I have always thought we were on to something, even though we don't have the proof-of-cause research yet.

Dioxins may also reduce the receptivity of endometrial cells to progesterone, which would certainly explain why progesterone support is needed, even though these women, in theory, can make it on their own[61]. Dioxins are a reportable chemical of sorts, and most governments have published the dioxin content of foods. If you search Dioxins on Health Canada or other government health agencies, you will see the amount of each type of food. The overwhelming theme is that it accumulates in animal-fat tissue; so animal products have the most. I used to advocate for a vegan diet for women with endometriosis. Truthfully, I don't know if we need to go that far. Some women get benefit from reducing the saturated fat in their diet and can keep the animal protein if they keep their choices limited to chicken, turkey and fish.

Observationally we see that women who eat more meat, and consume fewer vegetables have more endometriosis[62,63]. It is unclear if this is related to the dioxin discussion, or if it also illustrates a relative imbalance between inflammation and anti-inflammatory foods (similar to the oxidative stress discussion in the LPD chapter). Your overall diet strategy should be to use anti-inflammatory oils (avocado, olive oil, nuts), lots of fish[64], and lots of fruits and vegetables. Skip the alcohol and soy protein[65,66] should only be included in the diet in modest amounts.

There are a couple of low-powered studies that show that very early exposure to soy, in childhood may increase the risk for endometriosis[67]. Remember you are not in that population because you already have it. So, I'd focus on the data on women with existing disease: soy is safe and beneficial.

OTHER CONSIDERATIONS

The other consideration for endometriosis depends on how you are primarily being treated. If you are in the midst of long course cycle suppression, then perhaps your other treatments are mostly to help you with your chemical-menopause-induced side effects. If you are struggling with your pain and quality of life since coming off the pill, you may need some of these other treatments to feel better until you get pregnant.

There is a bit of a myth that you shouldn't be on any hormonal or anti-hormonal therapy before you try and get pregnant. When I see "natural" or "integrative" practitioners trying to recommend a drug detox to women before they try and get pregnant my response is always the same—they are not working with sick enough women. What I mean by that is if you truly understood the level of pain and inflammation in women with endometriosis, you'd respect the hell out of the disease. You'd never suggest doing a treatment that lowered control of lesions, and you would have looked it up in the research, and found that Lupron for 3-6 months before IVF may improve outcomes. You don't need a drug detox if you have severe disease. The only circumstance that I'd recommend coming off your drugs is if your goal is to come off your medications. Discontinuing your primary therapy may not help you get pregnant or stay pregnant, but if you feel deep in your soul that drug therapy is wrong, then by all means.

The problem with the medications for endometriosis is that they chemically turn off your hormones, which makes women menopausal. With that comes all of the lovely side effects such as hot flashes, insomnia and vaginal dryness. Long-term, the consequences of these drugs are problematic such as bone loss and heart disease risk but for fertility purposes, being on a shorter course likely does not cause dramatic long-term effects.

Hormonal add-back therapy is a slippery slope. We don't want your quality of life ruined by your drug therapy, but we also want it to work. There have been multiple studies on add-back treatment for endometriosis, but none of them has specifically looked at the 3-6 months before a fertility procedure. I would recommend to try and tolerate the side effects or try one of the more natural suggestions below. Only if you really cannot tolerate the treatment, and you have months to go, would a minimal dose of estrogen topically be indicated. There are target levels of blood estrogen to keep you below to prevent regrowth of your endometriosis. We think if we keep you below 100-150 pmol/L (30-40 pg/mL) on blood measures of estrogen we are not at risk for ruining the treatment[68]. But remember, this is from women expected to be on Lupron long term for their disease, not in women we are trying to prep for fertility. I don't know if adding back estrogen when you are getting ready for an IVF cycle is a good idea. I'd play it on the safe side and say no, unless your drug-induced menopause is too much to handle.

Resveratrol is the grape antioxidant, which is also in red wine, and has been shown to suppress endometriosis-related growths after surgery. CAUTION with this one: it has been shown to lower the effect of your Lupron or GnRH inhibitor drug. If you are doing a short or long course cycle suppression program before your IVF, you CANNOT take resveratrol at the same time. I think this is the only drug-nutrient interaction in this entire book and points out the importance of having a practitioner work with you on your treatment plan. The place for resveratrol is to improve antioxidant capacity, but also to prevent regrowth after surgery. It is a fertility-sparing option for women who don't want to do Lupron—or for women who cannot tolerate the side effects.

Black cohosh is an excellent option for your night sweats and hot flashes induced by your drug therapy while you prep for your IVF cycle[69]. Studies have compared it head to head against commonly used drugs, and it works just as well, with fewer side effects. It is a massive myth that black cohosh exerts an estrogen-like force. It will not cause regrowth of your lesions. We even use it in breast cancer patients with estrogen-positive tumors. If that cannot convince you, I don't know what else to say.

ENDOMETRIOSIS AND DRUGS

So, unless your goal is to get pregnant the most natural way possible, if you have endometriosis, your best bet is likely to combine both the conventionally offered treatments (surgery or drugs), nutrients and diet support as well as IVF.

Now I'm not saying you are doomed to use advanced reproductive technology (ART). Not at all. The severity of endometriosis in every woman is the predictor of her success. It is not a "yes you have it and therefore you must" situation. There are algorithms to help us determine what to do with you based on where your spots are, how large they are if they have caused scaring etc. These might help you make some decisions.

The gist of surgery is: if we think it will reduce uterine adhesions or structural changes in severe endometriosis then we should likely do it. If you have endometriosis on the ovary, we run some risk of damaging it if we try and take it out. Risk-benefit needs to be looked at here. *Are you in agony? Can you work? Is one ovary clear and one affected?* Talk to your surgeon. I generally find specialists who work specifically on endometriosis to be some of the most compassionate and integrative doctors out there. They work with women in pain every day and have your best interest in mind when it comes to fertility.

As for drugs, the current recommendation, in my opinion, is to do long-course suppression of your cycle before your IVF. Long course suppression can cause regression of some lesions, relieve your pain, and lets some of the inflammation dissolve before you try and get pregnant. Women who do long-course suppression have better IVF success and less miscarriage than women who do a shorter course, or who are not suppressed before IVF at all[53]. I cannot match that with anything natural, so again, think about what your goals are. I'm just telling you the facts.

Progesterone for endometriosis should be considered for every month as you prepare for your pregnancy unless you are doing drug therapy to suppress your cycle before an IVF. Women with short cycles are at a higher risk for endometriosis. Interestingly in most studies, they define a 'short' cycle as anything equal or less than 27 days[70]. Truthfully that's well within the range of 'normal' that we expect to see in the population, but if your cycle is short, progesterone may help improve the length while we work on lowering inflammation. One of the cooler studies on progesterone for endometriosis was trying to look at inflammation, and uterine tissue structure in women supplemented with progesterone, and they found better immune function and less inflammation but also noticed an improvement in egg quality and other markers of fertility. Their IVF cycles were more successful than they expected them to be, and the miscarriage rate was only 16%, which is technically lower than we expect[71]. There was no control group in the study, so we cannot say without a doubt that it helped them not miscarry. The nuances of science! But, based on the cycle benefits and immune benefits, I would recommend progesterone for women with endometriosis.

PROGESTERONE RECOMMENDATIONS FOR ENDOMETRIOSIS

* Progesterone suppositories day 14 to 28 of each cycle, or from the day of your fertility treatment until the day you have a confirmed viable pregnancy or are considered at low risk for miscarriage (9-12 weeks).

The evidence is pointing towards us using progesterone from ovulation or the day of oocyte transfer, until at least seven weeks of gestation. This is the protocol currently being studied in women with endometriosis, although we don't have enough results yet to say whether or not it helps. I suspect that we would see fewer miscarriage rates in women who do progesterone, but it may not undo months of inflammation without being used as part of a complete plan. (The women in the study did not use long-course GnRH inhibitors for example, which I would recommend).

HIGH HOMOCYSTEINE

So, I'm guessing you have never even heard the word homocysteine before reading this book, and I'm sitting here telling you this is a primary cause of miscarriage in women.

Homocysteine has created quite a stir in the miscarriage research world. We used to think it was a biomarker for some other problem. Meaning, if we found elevated levels, you must have a B12 deficiency or celiac disease. It was always viewed as a marker for some other problem. If we fixed the other problem, then the homocysteine would likely go away. The thing is, B12 deficiency does not cause miscarriage. The actual biomarker does. So rather than it being just a marker of something else, it has become its own thing[16]. Homocysteine is bad. So why are some women making so damn much of it?

Homocysteine is an amino acid (protein building block) that gets produced as an intermediate between two essential amino acids. As you make cysteine from methionine, homocysteine is briefly made in between. The problem lies in the arrows between methionine and cysteine. If you remember back to high school science, every reaction has arrows between them, and enzymes or nutrients that make those arrows work.

Between methionine and cysteine, there are arrows. And those arrows require good genetics and nutrients like B12 and folate. Fortunately, minimal amounts of B12 and folate lower homocysteine. This is good news because it is easy to treat, but bad news because even if you have been haphazardly taking your prenatal, you may have lowered your levels, and be masking your miscarriage diagnosis. Technically you are not at risk for miscarriage unless your levels are high, but if you had had a few miscarriages in the past when you were not taking a prenatal, you might be a high homocysteine girl, but your low dose B vitamins or multi-vitamin are going to hide it.

Homocysteine also increases in other ways, mostly as a downstream effect of obesity. Women who are overweight or who have PCOS make more homocysteine in their liver because of elevated insulin[72]. Insulin blocks an enzyme (fancily named cystathionine α synthetase) which prevents the breakdown of homocysteine, resulting in higher levels. This is also why women with PCOS are at an increased risk of heart disease as they age.

When homocysteine is elevated, for whatever reason, it directly disrupts placental development. Boom. Miscarriage. We have even in laboratory models where homocysteine causes uterine contractions in vitro[73]. So, you can see our big problem.

DIAGNOSIS

The testing for this is relatively easy. We have to look at your homocysteine level when you have fasted. Technically B12 and folate status can be tested as well, but regardless of how good those numbers look, if your homocysteine is high, you need those nutrients in higher amounts than you currently take in. Risks of going into your pregnancy with high homocysteine — if you don't miscarry — are preeclampsia, premature labour, premature rupture of membranes, and gestational diabetes[74]. Babies born in a high homocysteine environment are also at higher risk of neural tube defects, Down's Syndrome and heart defects[16]. Likely the challenges that present in babies are due to the genetic nature of homocysteine levels, so I also recommend that women who have carried to term before, but who's baby is afflicted with one of those conditions to get tested before her next pregnancy.

Unfortunately, we don't have a lot of signs and symptoms of elevated homocysteine. Most resources cite fatigue as being the most prominent symptom.

PHYSICAL SYMPTOMS OF WHICH MAY INDICATE HIGH HOMOCYSTEINE

* Increased waist circumference, elevated BMI or obesity.
* Physical symptoms associated with PCOS that can be found in the PCOS section.

LABORATORY MARKERS FOR HIGH HOMOCYSTEINE

* Elevated fasted homocysteine levels
* B12 levels below 200 pmol/L
* Elevated fasting Insulin (>50 pmol/L) , and other diagnostic measures for PCOS.

OTHER TESTING CONSIDERATIONS

Having high homocysteine, whether related to your genetics, a vitamin deficiency or PCOS causes vascular inflammation and increases your risk of cardiovascular disease. I would suggest doing some additional tests to look at your heart disease risks such as a cholesterol panel, CRP and any other markers associated with heart disease that your primary practitioner would be willing to run.

We are learning a lot every year about how our genetics are dictating our nutritional needs, and folic acid has taken the stage in the last few years as a point of interest. Every woman knows that folic acid is essential, but not every woman knows that her genetics dictate how "usable" the folate she consumes is. When we eat plain old folate from food or a supplement, we need our bodies to activate it into usable folate or methyltetrahydrofolate – I know, quite a mouthful. The ability to do this well or not depends on an enzyme MTHFR or methyltetrahydrofolate reductase. If you cannot activate folate, you cannot get rid of homocysteine. See the problem?

Currently, the studies don't suggest we test women for MTHFR genetic deficiencies[26,75] and in my ten years of practice, I have never checked it. Lots of my colleagues do, but I'm curious as to what they are doing with the results different than what I'm about to suggest. Remember that a lab needs to tell us something we don't already know (okay so testing your MTHFR status would do that) but, it also has to change the treatment. The treatment for these women is to take activated folate instead of plain folate. I think I can make a case that we should do this in all women anyways, so save the hundreds you'd spend on the test and get an excellent prenatal vitamin.

The treatment for this is straightforward. We need to fix the arrows between cysteine and methionine.

TREATMENT CONSIDERATIONS

Reducing homocysteine is really about making specific chemical processes more efficient. We know you cannot move from point A to point B without taking a detour at point H (homocysteine). So, we will add more fuel to the car, and that will take you there. You will continue to make some H likely, but if we give your body all of the nutrients, at least the potential to get to point B is there.

The studies that have looked at supplementation have done it with such incredibly low doses for the most part. I will explain what they did, then tell you what I think. I'm mostly recommending slightly higher doses because we are not doing a massive investigation to find out why your such-and-such vitamin is low. So, without harm, you should be taking a therapeutic dose, not just the bare minimum to lower a biomarker. With me? If you have elevated homocysteine because your B12 is low, getting you off the bottom of the reference range won't fix your fatigue. If you have high homocysteine because you have MTHFR issues, just giving you enough folate to lower your homocysteine may not reduce your risk of having a baby with a neural tube defect. So here we go.

SUPPLEMENT CONSIDERATIONS FOR HIGH HOMOCYSTEINE

* Folic Acid (Methylfolate type) 1-5 mg depending on your risk. Folate over 1 mg is a prescription in many jurisdictions. Talk to your practitioner if you need more than 1 mg[76,77]
* B12 (Methylcobalamin type) at least 400-5000 mcg, depending on your lab work and other symptoms.

Folate is the crutch of the process. Folic acid is a long-discussed nutrient in pregnancy ever since we figured out that by supplementing in women trying to conceive, we could reduce the risk of neural tube defects, heart defects and other congenital problems.

Enter mass folate-fortified flour phase.

Maybe this is news to you, but the government is giving you folate. Flour fortification of folate seems to fly under the radar (whereas everyone knows about iodine in salt) and as a public health initiative has likely improved birth outcomes on the whole. But what if you cannot make the folate into MTHF? What if the minuscule doses you get in flour are not enough for you? What if you are on a low carb diet? What if you are gluten-free? All fair questions I think.

Given that there is an inactive and an active type of folic acid, I think it is safe to assume that we should skip over the dollar store version of a nutrient and go with the top-shelf option. I hope you agree.

The evidence generally agrees with us. MTHF increases folic acid levels faster in women who haven't supplemented before, and by taking plain old folate[77], it can take 12-24 weeks to get your blood levels high enough to protect your baby. Even my most type A women are not usually supplementing that long before they hope to conceive. MTHF can increase your levels in a couple of weeks.

Vitamin B12 is also necessary to lower homocysteine and is very commonly deficient in women. It is not that abundant in our diet (milk, egg yolks, red meat) and as a result of our vegetarians and vegans need to supplement. As a funny aside, at one time we thought vegans had heart disease risk because their homocysteine was high. It was just their low B12 status.

B12 is also not easy to absorb, so it is often deficient in women with celiac, inflammatory bowel disease, or IBS just from poor absorption. The studies use very low dose B12 to lower homocysteine, so as long as its Methyl B12 the amount you get in your prenatal is likely enough. There are multiple forms of B12 and the studies often use 'lesser' quality B12 to get their results. I suggest you go top-shelf again and use the methylated B12 to get the most out of your support. Also, now that I'm on my soapbox and have a captive audience, you should still have your B12 tested, especially if you're tired or depressed.

Other supplements such as B6 have crept their way into homocysteine-lowering protocols over the years, but truthfully, they don't do much, and there is no evidence they lower miscarriage. Stick with the good stuff.

DIETARY RECOMMENDATIONS FOR HIGH HOMOCYSTEINE

* Increase sources of betaine in the diet[78,79]
* Increase sources of choline in the diet[80]
* Diet adjustments to achieve lower fasting insulin and weight loss.

Betaine is a nutritional molecule (sourced most often from beets, hence the name "bet") that also lowers homocysteine. I have discussed how to include betaine in your pre-pregnancy diet in the fertility diet section. Increasing betaine in the diet has been shown to be as effective as supplementation for reducing Homocysteine, and since supplementing betaine has not been studied in pregnancy, let's stay on the safe side and eat it instead.

Choline has been found to increase betaine levels and may help lower homocysteine, although not as good as betaine itself. The reason I include this, even though the research is spotty, is that the benefits to your baby from a high choline diet are immense. I discuss this further in the diet section but is worth an honorable mention here too.

The other thing to consider with elevated homocysteine is the role of your weight. Homocysteine goes up as weight increases, even if your B12 and folate status are picture perfect. Remember, in addition to being a nutrient-dependent thing; Homocysteine is also a marker of metabolic and cardiovascular disease. Weight loss is a beneficial way of reducing Homocysteine levels in non-pregnant patients, so I would consider the role of carrying around extra weight on your Homocysteine too. Women with PCOS who are obese have higher Homocysteine than non-obese PCOS women (and both are higher than non-PCOS women). A lower-carb weight loss plan that supports 0.5 to 1 pound of weight loss per week is a sustainable way of both losing weight and lowering Homocysteine.

OTHER CONSIDERATIONS

This section is mostly about monitoring once you do finally get and stay pregnant. Women who have tested positive for high homocysteine before should be observed closely given that they have a high likelihood of developing a high-risk pregnancy. Almost every pregnancy complication, from pre-eclampsia to premature labour have been linked to homocysteine levels. If you ever once test positive, I want you watched very carefully in your pregnancy. Don't shrug off swelling, minor blood pressure increases or protein in your urine. Each signals that you need more medical attention. Be sure your obstetrician or midwife knows your history.

HASHIMOTO'S (AUTOIMMUNE) THYROIDITIS

Thyroid dysfunction in early pregnancy is a soap opera of controversy. I dive into this in more detail later, but here are a few stumbling blocks that leave me scratching my head;

* If we universally test women for low thyroid and antibodies, we find out that a lot of women have problems but no symptoms ("Subclinical")[15]
* Women with low thyroid or antibodies (notice the "or", this is important) have between two and 10 x the miscarriage rates of women with normal thyroid function[14]
* If we treat women with low thyroid or antibodies, we reduce the frequency of miscarriage[81,82].
* Most societies have published position statements against universal screening.

Make sense to you? Me neither.

Technically for something to be considered a useful screening test it should be cheap, reliable, dramatically impact outcomes, have easy and accessible treatment options etc. There are prominent authors in the field who have written in support of universal screening for low thyroid and miscarriage and remind everyone that the only way we have come to learn as much as we know about thyroid dysfunction and miscarriage is through studies that universally screened women and then treated them. So, don't get caught in the drama. Population screening politics shouldn't get in the way of you being tested. I routinely check all women who are thinking about getting pregnant for low thyroid. I universally screen you.

YOUR THYROID GLAND IN PREGNANCY

Pregnancy is a bit of a wild ride for your thyroid, and if things are perfectly healthy, the transient stress and changes to the thyroid economy are not a problem. Hormone levels go up and down, proteins that bind these hormones to go up and down, and in a healthy woman the net result is zero change. You carry on, your hormones don't become a problem, and you carry to term. If, anywhere in those 10 steps you have a problem, like in iodine deficiency—which is very uncommon in Canada, but still prevalent in many European countries—or if your thyroid was a bit stressed before you got pregnant, these subtle shifts can change your hormone levels enough to put you into a state of hypothyroidism, and this causes miscarriage.

You need your thyroid to rise to the occasion of pregnancy. If the underlying resources or thyroid reserve is not there, it cannot. Even stimulated IVF cycles are technically stress on the thyroid. If you have had multiple failed IVF cycles with no identified cause, I'd like to see you tested for antibodies before you go through another stimulated cycle.

Even if you are already on medication for your thyroid, we need to be paying close attention. About 80% of women who are already medicated will require a dose adjustment very early in pregnancy. The other 20% were likely over-medicated before they got pregnant[14]. Not a problem necessarily, I only say this because it highlights that even in 'treated' women, we need to be paying close attention to your lab work to make sure that your thyroid stays in good control. It is crucial that you get lab work done regularly and that your dose changes are monitored until your numbers get into the ideal range. Some women need a frank doubling of their medication amount, while some can get by with a small increase. We find out by testing, so be sure that you go.

What we are not entirely sure of is why autoimmune thyroid/Hashimoto's Thyroid (HT) or hypothyroid without antibodies cause miscarriage. Technically the real issues with the thyroid and pregnancy get worse as you go along. Yes, early gestation sees some shifts in thyroid function, but most of the significant changes to hormone levels are observed as we move through trimester two and three, so it cannot entirely account for why we see increased miscarriage in women with low thyroid.

The autoimmune aspect might explain it for women who have tested positive for TPO. Women with all autoimmune disease are at risk for miscarriage, and women with other autoimmune disease are at an increased risk of Hashimoto's antibodies as well. If you have type 1 diabetes or celiac, I insist that you get screened. If you have another different autoimmune disease, it is likely a good idea too.

The big take home is to get screened, even if you are asymptomatic. We are trying to be proactive here, so let's not wait until you have had multiple miscarriages before we test you. Hypothyroid women face complications during their pregnancy such as fetal growth restriction, hypertension, premature delivery and fetal hypothyroidism, so even if the problem is not enough to miscarry, it can become a problem further down the line if left unaddressed[83,84].

CHAPTER 4 — THE DIAGNOSIS

DIAGNOSING HASHIMOTO'S

If you want to watch a Naturopath and a Medical Doctor fight, give them some lab work with a TSH (thyroid stimulating hormone) of 3.5 mIU/L. I have had the good fortune of working with the family medical resident teams at my local hospital on integrative care models. The only thing we fight about is TSH. Fertility is a fantastic example of how thyroid function is supposed to go, and how we should be valuing it more in the general population. Always remember: we need your body to be functioning correctly to get pregnant. If you keep this in mind, the rest becomes easy. Sort of.

So here are some things we notice in the research: if women have autoimmune thyroiditis — elevated antibodies against their thyroid — their TSH needs to be below 2.5 to get pregnant.

So, let's put that all together. The body must function optimally. TSH in some women needs to be below 2.5 to get pregnant. Why then, is the reference range for TSH up to 4.0. What is happening to those women between 2.5 and 4? Take a wild guess. They struggle with their weight, they are tired, and they cannot get pregnant. I have watched women get pregnant just by fixing this one number. Its importance in fertility cannot be underestimated.

Like I mentioned in the last section, I am in support of universally screening women who are looking to conceive for thyroid dysfunction. And so is the research. One review looked at measuring pre-conception women in the "old" way (only if you have a strong family history, are tired, or overweight) compared to just testing everyone. If they tested everyone, they found thyroid dysfunction twice as often[15]. Enough said. When you have a thyroid panel done, it indeed should consist of a few tests. You have probably only had your TSH tested at your annual physical. TSH is the conventional standard test, and interestingly public health is not too worried about the other four numbers. From a fertility perspective, the other numbers matter. You a full thyroid panel, which includes TSH, T4, T3 and antibody levels (TPO and anti-TG). You need all the tests.

The reason I put so much emphasis on the lab work is that physically you might not be able to tell if you have a low thyroid. We often think about tired, overweight women with hair loss, cold hands and trouble concentrating. And although this is all true, it is sub-clinical (meaning you have no symptoms) hypothyroid that is probably getting in the way of making babies. This is why we need the tests. I also would put a lot of emphasis on the lab work if you have any other autoimmune disease (including Celiac) or have any of the other conditions talked about in this book (including APS, and PCOS) since the chances of having thyroid antibodies are higher in these groups of women.

PHYSICAL SIGNS OF HASHIMOTO'S THYROIDITIS

* Weight gain or difficulty managing your weight
* Fatigue
* Muscle or joint pains

- ✱ Constipation or slow digestion
- ✱ Difficulty maintaining body temperature (always cold)
- ✱ Thinning or dry hair
- ✱ Low mood

LABORATORY SIGNS OF HASHIMOTO'S THYROIDITIS

- ✱ TSH elevated above 2.0 (some texts want below 1-1.5 mIU/L for optimal fertility)
- ✱ T4 and T3 (the goal should be around 50% of the reference range or greater)
- ✱ TPO (Thyroid Peroxidase) is an autoantibody that if positive, will lower chances of a successful pregnancy.
- ✱ Anti-TG (Thyroglobulin) is another antibody that if positive, means you have an autoimmune low thyroid.
- ✱ Vitamin D levels are correlated to antibody levels and are part of the treatment for HT.

For future, even if you don't have low thyroid right now, you should be retested six weeks and six months postpartum. A significant number of women develop thyroid antibodies after pregnancy and should be tested and treated accordingly.

TREATMENT CONSIDERATIONS

The significant treatment for autoimmune hypothyroid is with hormone replacement therapy, but in addition to that, we find if we can lower the thyroid antibodies in women with HT then we can improve her fertility outcomes and help reduce the risk of miscarriage. Even after getting pregnant, women with elevated TPO (antibodies) have an increased risk of pregnancy complications, so we likely want to focus on this anyways, even if you have successfully made it through the first trimester.

SUPPLEMENT CONSIDERATIONS FOR HASHIMOTO'S THYROIDITIS

* Selenium 200 mcg per day as selenomethionine[85,86]
* Vitamin D to treat your deficiency[87]

DIETARY RECOMMENDATIONS FOR HASHIMOTO'S THYROIDITIS

* Check your iodine intake and adjust it if necessary[88]
* Avoid gluten if you have also tested positive for celiac

There are a lot of "thyroid support" supplements out there with herbs and nutrients intended to support thyroid function. None of them has had any research for HT beyond selenium and vitamin D, and the use of these nutrients is limited to improving your antibody levels. We don't even have an excellent study that shows that they reduce the risk of miscarriage. We want your antibodies to be lower, although we are not clear whether the early miscarriage in women with HT is related to the autoimmune side of the disease, or the low thyroid side of the disease. So, we work to lower antibodies anyways. This is an excellent holistic way of thinking about your condition. You have inflammation and immune dysfunction, that's a bad thing for miscarriage, so we will work on lowering it.

We used to have a significant iodine deficiency issue in North America, with goitres (visible growth of the thyroid) happening regularly right up until my grandma's generation. The government stepped in iodized salt, and voila. We no longer have a problem. Fast forward a few decades, and we find the populations that eat the most iodine are at the most at risk for autoimmune thyroid. Go figure. So even though we don't have any evidence that taking iodine out of the diet improves TPO, or miscarriage rates, I certainly would not go out of your way to eat a ton of extra of iodine. I'm always surprised at the number of women taking sea-vegetable products like kelp to "boost their metabolism". Stop. You don't need it, and it might be worsening the problem. Check your prenatal multi-vitamin. Your pregnancy goals for iodine is about 200 micrograms. In all likelihood, you are getting enough, but if you're worried about it, track your food and supplement sources to confirm.

The gluten-free diet should be prescribed and followed to a tee in women who have tested positive for celiac. The recommendation to follow a gluten-free diet has crept into the recommendations for women with HT. I'm not sure if this is because often women have both? Or if someone once somewhere got a few women with HT pregnant after following a gluten-free diet? The truth is, we don't have any evidence for it. Eating gluten-free makes everyone feel better. If it makes you feel better, then do it. If it doesn't, don't. Simple!

HORMONE AND DRUG SUPPORT

Medicating women trying to conceive who have tested positive for Hashimoto's is an essential part of the treatment. It is important that your practitioner is well versed and willing to prescribe thyroid hormone if you have tested positive for antibodies. If they are not, move on sister. We don't have time to play around. Over the last few years, the research has suggested we should be pushing TSH lower and lower in women with HT to achieve pregnancy, reduce miscarriage, and reduce complications during pregnancy. As a reminder, here's how that works.

TSH is made by your brain to stimulate your thyroid to produce thyroid hormone (T4). T4, after being made, signals back to your brain to stop making so much TSH. It is called a negative feedback loop. Your brain and thyroid keep talking to each other to tell each other how to be supported. As your thyroid gets worse at responding, your brain sends a stronger signal. Think of TSH going up as your brain slapping your thyroid across the face. So, we use TSH to watch how functional your thyroid is. If your brain is sending a stronger signal, your thyroid may not be listening, or it is trying to hear, but cannot seem to respond. Sounds like my kids.

So, although we let women who are not trying to get pregnant have a TSH in the 2.5-4 range and don't seem to care, women who are trying to conceive can improve their chances of success if we get them into a "more ideal" range. We are now medicating women with a completely normal hormone profile and finding we can get them pregnant. So, if your goals are to get pregnant at all costs, and you have lined yourself up for expensive reproductive technology, AND you have Hashimoto's thyroid, you need medication. STAT.

There are a few studies due out that refer to medicating women with HT who have a TSH below 3.5[81,82]. The preliminary results are finding that they can get pregnant easier if they are medicated with synthetic T4.

So, which form of thyroid hormone should you use?

There are two types of thyroid hormone replacement out there: synthetic T4 (LT4) and desiccated thyroid hormone (DT). LT4 is fake, made by a pharmaceutical company (often goes by the name Synthroid or Levothyroxine or Eltroxin) and DT is a natural source of thyroid hormone that comes from pork. DT has some positive studies in women with low thyroid, and it seems patients like it better, and they may lose more weight on it[89]. But read me loud and clear: we have no evidence to use this in pregnancy.

Natural is not always better, and DT might be a great example of this. The differences between LT4 and DT lie in the details. They have different ratios of T4/T3 which is often cited as the benefit of DT, with LT4 having no T3, and DT having a more natural ratio between the two hormones. Maybe in women who are not trying to get pregnant, this is a good thing, but when the only T4 crosses the placenta, adding T3 to the system may interfere with those feedback loops.

The American Thyroid Association admits that the statement to not use DT in pregnancy is based on weak evidence. But we don't have substantial evidence to use it either. We have hundreds of studies on LT4. Maybe thousands. Let's go with a low-risk medication that we have studied to death over the more natural version for now.

If you have been helped to get pregnant on DT, once you get pregnant you will want to switch to LT4. Simple solution. Once you start your medication, your TSH should be tested every six weeks until you're in the ideal range, less than 2.0, and then checked again after you deliver. In my experience, OB/GYN docs will only change your medication if your TSH gets very high and there is frank risk to the baby, but for optimal pregnancy support and to carry to term your primary practitioner should frequently monitor your lab work for you.

THE UNCOMMON BUT IMPORTANT CAUSES OF MISCARRIAGE

I have done my best to address the most critical areas for you to be investigated in if you have had recurrent miscarriage, but if you have been through each of the tests mentioned in the previous sections, and you are still "unexplained" you may want to seek some assessment for some of the more uncommon causes of miscarriage. Most of the leftover diagnoses are immune and blood clotting related, and truthfully the treatment does not change that much, even if we don't nail down the actual why of your miscarriages.

The challenges with the leftovers are that we don't have great assessment techniques to tell us what's going on. We know that women with any autoimmune disease have an increased risk of miscarriage and we know that women with recurrent miscarriage have different white blood cell counts in her uterus[90] but not necessarily in her blood, so we cannot measure it[91] with standard testing. Knowing either of these things does not help guide treatment. We use anticoagulants, progesterone and cross our fingers.

My hope for the future research in miscarriage is that we start to develop the understanding of women who fall into this category of 'unexplained' miscarriage better. I want better lab testing, better treatment options and a better understanding of how miscarriage from these causes affects a woman's total health. Each of the other causes of miscarriage is full-body conditions, and these likely are too, we just haven't spent time on it yet.

ANTIPHOSPHOLIPID SYNDROME (APS) is likely the most well understood 'leftover' diagnosis that I haven't covered yet. I have only seen it a handful of times in my clinical practice, most fertility clinics don't test for it, and the actual percentage of women who struggle with it is very low. The challenge with the diagnosis is that to qualify; you need to have had recurrent miscarriages in addition to testing positive for autoantibodies (anti-cardiolipin and anti-lupus antibody). The treatment includes anticoagulants such as aspirin, heparin and of course progesterone. There are a couple of papers out there that look at using fish oil instead of Aspirin in women with clotting issues and miscarriage[92]. I suggest fish oil in the supplement section for all women, so you should be covered.

CHAPTER 5

YOU ARE WHAT YOU EAT (AND WHAT YOU DON'T EAT)

When I first graduated I approached a big fertility clinic in town to talk to them about how to better help their patients prepare for their procedures and to present the evidence on how to improve their IVF statistics with diet. I admit I was young and optimistic at that time and was just thrilled that they had given me the lunchtime meeting—of which 80% of the doctors were late for. I wasn't booed off stage (although at the time it felt like it), but every scrap of evidence I presented that diet made an impact was met with so much criticism that I cried in my car in the parking lot after. True story.

So, what was this radical information that I shared? Well, I started with the data that a relatively large percentage of women in the month before their IVF (read: the biggest day of their year) still drink both alcohol, and caffeine. We also know very well that these things reduce the chances of successful implantation. The study suggested that maybe we don't do a great job of educating women about the things they can do in their last four weeks that might improve their odds. I presented a study with 120 patients that looked at how many women had "bad behavior" the few weeks before their procedure (I'm not judging, I'm paraphrasing)[93]. The doctors told me the study was too small, and that *their* patients behave better during the month of their IVF. Funnily enough, a few years later, the same author published a study with 12,800 women all across the United States and found the same thing[94]. Which makes me think their patients were not that different than the women studied.

I also presented on diet manipulation in women with PCOS, and how by eating a lot for breakfast and a little for dinner (even if we did not change the poor diet the women were eating) improved ovulation rates and fertility success rates by about 50%. Their response? "Our success is better than what's published in that study, so it was probably done at a terrible fertility clinic."

Wait a minute?

Forget the numbers for a second. Just telling your patients *when* to eat, might improve their success? And you're telling me that your ego is too big to consider talking to your patients about it? Or worse, your ego is too big to let me speak to them about it? These are thoughts I had after — as I dreamed up smart comebacks in my car. More tears.

The experience was very negative for me. I swore off a bunch of things after that day. No more meeting with

Doctors. No more educating Doctors. No more fertility care. And no more crying in my car in the parking lot. For God's sake Jordan at least drive away first.

So, does food have an impact?

Ten years later I can confidently say yes. I started treating fertility again in the last few years. But really, I did swear you all off for a short time there. I even hired a second doctor in my office to see you instead.

When I graduated Naturopathic Medical School, NDs were all about the radical diets. Gluten-free for everyone! Dairy is the devil! Brown rice lives! And this clashed with my real-life patient population. My fertility patients kept asking me if they could just quit coffee and alcohol from day 14 to day 28 (ovulation to fertilization) and if they did not get pregnant start drinking them again. I'm not kidding.

Now you, might feel slightly more ambitious than patients from my past. But my newly graduated brain mixed with this not-willing-to-sacrifice group of women made me feel a little frustrated over the whole thing. Then a funny thing happened. I spent ten years researching the topic.

The truth is, I think we can compromise a bit on the diet thing and focus on what matters rather than just making your life miserable for the sake of sacrifice. Yes, you'd feel better if you went gluten-free. Everyone does. Is it medically necessary for everyone? Maybe not. This should be about helping you get healthier than you are right now, not be the healthiest uterus on the planet. Can we shake on it?

> I solemnly promise to only present information that has real human clinical data on a diet, as long as you promise not to ask if you can do it for half the month. I'm hoping we have a deal.

ALCOHOL

I'm not trying to be your friend. I'm trying to get you pregnant and carry to term. So, what I'm about to say about alcohol and caffeine I'm speaking as a doctor. I'm going to be brutally honest—alcohol is getting in the way of you getting pregnant. Every which way we look at it, whether it is the female partner or the male, alcohol is a problem for fertility. It causes failed IUI/IVF cycles, and it causes miscarriage.

ALCOHOL CAUSES MISCARRIAGE

We don't get to use that word in medicine very often. "Cause". We sort of pussy-foot around causation most of the time because we never want to say things without a shadow of a doubt (because that's not how science works). The moment we say something causes something is the moment we start practicing belief-based medicine and stop evolving. I digress. But I'm perfectly willing, after the virtual-piles of articles I have read to say without a shadow of a doubt that alcohol causes miscarriage.

> *Still friends? Wait until we get to the caffeine section!*

The other thing that bites is that you can't have any — none. We cannot find a small amount that does not cause miscarriage. So, you're out of luck. If you want to justify a 1/2 glass of white wine in a spritzer that's up to you, but technically — according to the research — it reduces your chances of carrying to term.

For the sake of numbers, or in case you don't believe me, there was a study that looked at both male and female alcohol consumption in the four weeks leading up to their IVF procedure[95]. The women in the study who drank (at all) in the four weeks leading up to their big day had fewer eggs collected, were 2.8 times more likely to have a failed cycle and were 2.2 x more likely to miscarry. The male partners who drank (at all) were 2.2 x more likely to have a failed cycle and were 2.7 x more likely to miscarry after getting a positive pregnancy test. The increased risk was seen with all doses of alcohol (so even one drink), and the chance went up with increased dose – so the more they drank, the worse the outcome.

RECOMMENDATION: *Abstain from alcohol for 12 weeks before your procedure, or until you have a healthy baby.*

CAFFEINE

I'm a major caffeine addict. But that also means, I have spent hundreds of hours researching the health effects of caffeine. Usually, we have good news to share about caffeine and coffee—except for miscarriage. It might be the worst thing you can do.

I remember the day I found all of this out. I was in my favorite coffee shop on one of my non-clinical days drinking a turbo Americano and stumbled on a study that showed that even as little as 100 mg of caffeine in the week before an IVF increased the chances of miscarriage. I was drinking about 300 mg as I was reading the study.

I then—with my highly caffeinated brain—stormed through another dozen studies that confirmed and strengthened the statement.

CAFFEINE CAUSES MISCARRIAGE.

The thing about miscarriage, which I have already alluded to, is that *when* the miscarriage happens is an important piece for us to examine. Is it before implantation? After? As the placenta develops? These details can tell us the mechanism by which things cause miscarriage and help us target treatment. They have looked at the relationship between caffeine and miscarriage and have found that caffeine increases "*sina causea*" miscarriage, Latin for "no cause"[96].

These no-cause miscarriages tell us something. The egg was perfect, and the uterus was ideal, and the process would have gone on uninterrupted if it had not been for caffeine.

Caffeine takes a perfectly good fertilized egg and miscarries it. So, put down the coffee girl. Unsurprisingly, the other thing we find, is that there is a dose-dependent effect of caffeine. The more you drink, the worse it is[97].

RECOMMENDATION: *abstain from caffeine for four weeks before your ART procedure, or until you deliver a healthy baby.*

THE FERTILITY DIET

I'm the first to admit when the research on a topic is slim, and although we are spending more time on this topic than we did ten years ago, there still are not the proper trials I want to see with diet and miscarriage. It is a hard topic to study. If people eat "healthier", they also eat less. So, did they feel better (or not miscarry) because of the "healthfulness" of the food or because they were in caloric restriction? We may never know. Funnily some trials have tried to fix these problems by controlling for calories. I have even seen ridiculous add-back strategies like whipped cream to keep the weight on the people, but then we run into other obvious issues. So, although we have a few specific recommendations, we have gathered most of our insight about diet and fertility by watching women in their natural habitat and see who gets pregnant.

Keep in mind the data is not on reducing miscarriage — it is about improving birth rates.

THIS IS WHAT WE KNOW SO FAR

Be in a healthy BMI range. Women should be closer to their ideal body weight for optimal fertility. If you are overweight, discussing a weight loss strategy that keeps everything else in check with your practitioner is a good start. BMI is directly linked to miscarriage rates, even if you don't have PCOS or another underlying 'cause' of your miscarriages[6]. Being closer to an ideal BMI reduces inflammation, decreases insulin, creates less stress in your body and creates a better hormonal environment.

Weight loss is HARD. Which is why I suggest working with someone who can cater to your plan and your goals. I'm going to take a massive side-bar here and go on a rant about weight loss so forgive me and hear me out.

> If your goals are wishy-washy, then your plan can also be wishy-washy.

This is what I tell every single patient, fertility or not, who is interested in losing weight. If your goal is to lose 5 lbs. in the next year, great! Put less sugar in your coffee and walk around a bit more and I will see you in a year. If your goal is to lose 12 pounds in 12 weeks, suddenly every molecule of food you put in your mouth matters. Both weight loss plans are possible. The problem is that people want to lose 12 pounds in 12 weeks, but don't want to be accountable, or track their food. Or change their food-court lunch. Or not eat dinner until 9 pm. If the weight loss industry has done anything, it has ruined our expectations of weight loss and made it seem that we shouldn't have to work that hard for it to happen.

Ultimately, the diet that works is the diet you follow. Get real about your expectations and goals — sit down with someone who knows what they are doing and construct a plan. Ideally a 12-week plan at minimum. Anyone can do anything for a few days. A real diet needs consistency and self-love to carry you through it.

Okay, I'm done.

PROTEIN SOURCES MATTER. The more saturated fat in a woman's diet, the higher the risk for infertility. There is likely an underlying hormonal issue here, given that high-fat foods can increase estradiol (and weight if you're not careful). Although you need at least a gram of protein per kilo of body weight, where you get that protein from is essential, and even replacing 5% of your high-fat animal protein with vegetarian protein can improve fertility. Perhaps as much as 50%[98].

Leaner proteins such as poultry and fish, protein powder and eggs are all great and very dense sources of protein. Keep beef, pork, lamb and bison for less frequent use. As popular as bacon is these days, it is not the best choice for my fertility gals. If you're not a meat-eating girl, you need to be even more mindful about adequate protein and be sure to have your iron tested somewhere along this journey.

Supplementing iron in women, in general improves their fertility[99].

Dairy is a thorn in my side. I have spent most of the last ten years worrying about its impact on endometriosis, PCOS and acne. In the best cohort study, we have on diet and fertility they suggested full-fat dairy over low-fat dairy[100] Here's what I would recommend. If you don't have acne, or PCOS, or endometriosis, then you can use dairy. Use whatever-fat seems to help you manage your protein and appetite the best. If high protein/low fat leaves you satisfied and helps maintain weight, great. If you need the full fat to increase your calories and make you feel full—great.

TRANS-FATS KILL, FISH-FATS DON'T. Trans-fats (margarine, bakery products, donuts, crackers, microwave popcorn) are not natural. They are made from the processing of other fats and have been straight up associated with an increased risk of death. It turns out that for every 2% of your healthy fats (olive oil) that is replaced with trans fats, it nearly doubles your risk of certain types of infertility[101]. Although they have not been directly linked with miscarriage, I don't think we need to wait for the study to make the recommendation. Just for the number's sake, that could be as low as a few grams of trans fats per day causing problems with your fertility. On the flip side, healthy fats have a positive role, especially omega-3 fats found in fish.

A Mediterranean style diet also has a positive impact on fertility in general[102], which uses mostly olive oil and fats found in nuts. If you are overweight, increasing dietary sources of omega 3s have been shown to improve your success rates with IVF. Choose a variety of dietary omega-3s such as fish, flax and hemp.

CARBS: ARE THEY FRIEND OR FOE? Now here's where it gets dicey. I cannot make a good carbohydrate recommendation across the board. Mostly because so many causes of miscarriage are related to weight and insulin. If you have a known issue with insulin and PCOS, you should be working with a practitioner who knows how to manipulate your diet to get the best outcome. Some women need 40% carbohydrate diets (40% of their total calories from carbs), some need less. You deserve a tailored plan.

Interestingly when we step back from miscarriage and look at fertility in general, total carbohydrate intake may not have a huge impact, but the TYPE of carbs may be playing the more significant role[103]. Even in my women with PCOS, we can see improvements with slight changes to higher fiber, lower glycemic foods (remember my high fiber melba toast example). The only carb that was a complete no-no according to the research was cold cereal.

So, here are my recommendations: no cold cereal. Ever. Unless you like eating your full flake oats cold occasionally. Also, replace every carb with the healthier version of itself. Replace white with brown, brown with browner, and try and increase your vegetables and legumes in place of your grain-based products. They carry with them more nutrition and help balance blood sugar better than bread.

MEET BETAINE & CHOLINE, YOUR NEW FRIENDS. Five supplements improve health outcomes in infants, one of which most women have never heard of: choline. Betaine and choline are cousins (choline is the precursor for betaine), and both have been shown to lower homocysteine. Choline improves neurological health in babies, especially when born into families with a strong history like schizophrenia or bipolar disorder. In the labs' section, we went over homocysteine, and it is role causing major interference in placental development.

Whether your fasting homocysteine is high or not, all women getting prepped for pregnancy could benefit from including high dietary sources of betaine and choline into their lives, to reduce their risk of miscarriage, and improve the health of their baby — which is why I have included it here. Betaine can be supplemented, but it has not been well studied enough in pregnancy for me to comment on it. I'd focus on food instead, as there is research saying it is just as good as the supplement anyways[78]. As for choline, you can supplement it safely if none of the foods fit your palate, or if you are vegan. Vegans and vegetarians are naturally low in choline and should consider a supplement to make up the difference during preconception. When we randomly survey all pregnant women, meat-eating or not, their intake is about half of what's ideal for the healthiest baby.

BETAINE CONTAINING FOODS
- Beets
- Chickpeas
- Grapefruit, orange
- Spinach
- Chicken
- Mussels
- Wheat flour
- Pasta
- Rolled Oats

CHOLINE CONTAINING FOODS
- Eggs
- Dairy
- Fish
- Chicken
- Turkey
- Pasta
- Rice
- Soy Lecithin (health food)
- Shrimp

Including more of these foods that naturally contain betaine and choline can reduce homocysteine and improve the health of your baby without adding supplements. If your measured homocysteine is high, then I would also suggest supplementing some of the nutrients found in the next sections (B12, Folate).

CHAPTER 6

STRESS AND EXERCISE

I have lumped these two beauties of a topic together for a good reason. They both cause anovulatory infertility in similar ways, and unfortunately we are just starting to understand a bit more about how they contribute to miscarriage.

Stress is in the eye of the beholder.

Stress is hard to study. We know that women who report more financial or personal stress after conceiving have more miscarriage. We also know that women who test high on validated personal life stress quizzes also have a higher rate of miscarriage. We know that women who have elevated levels of cortisol (the stress hormone) after conceiving also miscarry upwards of 90% of the time, and we know that if a woman's stress hormone goes up after conceiving (or IVF), she is also more likely to miscarry[25].

Did I stress you out?

The problem with stress is that we don't always find elevated stress hormones AND elevated quiz results in the same women. Sometimes the quiz is high, and the hormone is low, sometimes the hormone is high, and the quiz is low. So now what the hell do we do? We have two ways of measuring stress, and they both seem to cause miscarriage. But they both might be positive in two different sets of women. This has made it hard to make a good connection between miscarriage and stress because the blood marker and the quiz results don't connect.

However, if either of them is high, we have a problem. I'm not sure we need large studies with thousands of women to conclude that stress is a problem for the generation of women currently trying to get pregnant. It is preventing us from ovulating in the first place, and then if we finally have our eggs meet a sperm, we miscarry more frequently.

Because we have had such a difficult time assessing it, we also don't have any science to show us what to do with you. Lowering cortisol and trying to reduce miscarriage would be a neat study. Meditation and stress management support to minimize miscarriage would also be a cool study. We haven't looked at either.

There are tools to reduce both, the perception of stress mentally, and your biological response to it. I would suggest taking a good look at your stress, have your cortisol tested, and come up with a plan to work in this area of your health. Meditation, walking outside, psychological support and acupuncture can support mental health in unique ways to lower the perception of psychological stress. The physical demands of stress can also be augmented by specific nutrition, supplements like fish oil, B complex and phospholipids like choline and phosphatidylserine.

I don't recommend grabbing any "adrenal" support off the shelf to treat yourself. Get tested and talk to someone who can formulate a pregnancy-safe plan. Many over the counter support act very much like drugs and may interact with your fertility plan.

Anyone can work on their mental health by lowering their perception of stress, focusing on what matters, and cultivating a life and relationships that bring joy and peace. Funnily, some of the bad science on acupuncture and fertility is likely because of the added stress of medical appointments. Women who had to travel to their acupuncture appointments had less success with their IVF than women who do it in-house at their fertility clinic—food for thought? Your fertility treatment plan shouldn't bring more stress, and I always offer acupuncture only if connecting with me and coming to my office gives the perception of less stress and more support.

EXERCISE IS ALL ABOUT BLOOD FLOW

Who better to comment on the connection between exercise and miscarriage than the International Olympic Committee? They have been tracking fertility and miscarriage in athletes for ages and have some great insight into what the problems are, and how to avoid them.

When we exercise we divert blood away from our internal organs, towards our muscles. It is been studied well in non-pregnant women, and as you move towards your maximal heart rate (or working at 75% or more) blood starts to shift to support your exercise. Makes sense doesn't it?

So, when we are trying our best to create a network of blood flow on a microscopic level to develop optimal placental health, diverting blood flow away from that project may not be the best idea. They have found that women who exercise intensely 7+ hours a week are at an increased risk of miscarriage[104]. The chance may be up to 3.5 times more than non-exercisers. Which is a lot.

Now in all seriousness, most of my patients are not elite athletes. However, per cent exertion is based on your body, so if you reach that 70% maximal output going for a steep walk, then you need to slow down. But not for long. It turns out that past the 20-week mark there was no difference in miscarriage rates between exercisers and non-exercisers. So, you have to scale back for a little while. If your regular exercise is below that 70% threshold, then keep at it. Exercise is good.

Lifting weight has been associated with increased miscarriage when it is part of a woman's job (so lifting a lot, all day long) so the IOC has suggested similar things concerning heavy load weightlifting. Wait a bit, and then it is probably okay.

Now even the IOC admits that we haven't spent enough time or resources studying this particular issue but taking a few weeks off heavy exercise never hurt anyone and may improve your success carrying to term. I'm pretty sure if I told you to stand on your head every day you'd do it, so walk, do yoga, or exercise below 70%.

CHAPTER 7
NUTRITIONAL SUPPLEMENTS

I'm always amazed by the shopping bags full of supplements people bring into their first appointment. Many patients self-prescribe, without ever having discussed their condition with a healthcare practitioner. "So and so" at the health food store only knows what the supplement companies have taught them (trust me, I worked in a health food store during my four years of my ND degree). Your well-intentioned relatives only know what the latest health blogger has written. It is a problematic war we wage with supplements being available over the counter. Yes, you can buy them and take them. But should you?

If you ever hear someone utter the phrase "natural medicine does not work" it is generally because they have taken a sub-therapeutic dose of glucosamine for their undiagnosed 'arthritis', and it did not magically go away in 2 weeks. These are my face-palming FML moments in my career. I have dedicated my life to researching integrative care, and newspaper headlines about bad products and anecdotes from people who were never assessed, who's supplements 'did not work' taint the public opinion of the entire field of integrative medicine.

The purpose of your supplements should be evident. Check your medicine cabinet, kitchen counter and bedside table. What are you taking? And maybe more importantly, why? The dose is essential, as is the form/type, time of day, and whether it is taken with food.

It sounds an awful lot like a prescription doesn't it?

The next section is going to focus on the supplements that have evidence for reducing miscarriage in the population we have been discussing in each of the earlier chapters. You will see that a few of the nutrients have reared their head in multiple spots and that a few of them are very condition specific. I have included them all in one section here for you to read about them all at once. No, you don't take them all. You don't need them all. So, do me a huge favour and don't read to the end and think to yourself, "I might as well just take them all and reduce my risk as much as possible". That's missing the point.

You know how I'd feel about that. I have purposefully mentioned which nutrients are right for each condition here, and in each condition-specific section for reference. Between the labs, explanation of your diagnosis and supplements you should have quite a list going of what to focus on.

CHAPTER 7 — NUTRITIONAL SUPPLEMENTS

SUPPLEMENTS, SUPPLEMENTS FOR EVERYONE

Now, I don't like to make assumptions. So, we are going to start with the absolute basics that you should be taking for optimal fertility and healthy pregnancy. We have done studies on women going for IVF, and you know what? Lots of them still drink. Most of them still have coffee. And a few of them even use recreational drugs. So, what does this mean? It means that we shouldn't assume you know what you're doing, and so here I have included a chapter on the basics of supplementation for a healthy pregnancy and optimal fertility.

The caveat here is that none of these supplements has been well studied concerning miscarriage. Yes, a multivitamin improves fertility; we don't think it reduces miscarriage. So, we are a bit off topic, but I cannot ignore the essential supplements that you should be taking to get pregnant in the first place.

In a major observational study, where they tracked thousands of women over a period of many years who were looking to get pregnant, they observed both the dietary and supplemental behaviours that seemed to help women get pregnant more often. And this is what they found.

YOU NEED A MULTI-VITAMIN (WITH ACTIVATED FOLIC ACID)

Multivitamins for pregnancy and fetal development are a significant milestone and step forward as far as reducing the risk of congenital developmental disorders. They reduce cardiovascular abnormalities and neurological defects. This was a significant win as far as medicine is concerned. A simple, inexpensive intervention that has essential outcomes for public health.

Now, I never recommend that my patients shoot for the public health level of health. Public health is meant to treat the masses. It is intended to reduce the most amounts of death and disability and to cost the government less in healthcare spending. All good things! But, if we look at what YOU want, it is not likely about doing the most good for the most people. It is about doing the most good for you. So, your recommendations may need to be different, and your standards for a multivitamin should, therefore, be different.

A major observational study, when tracking fertility in thousands of women, over almost a decade, found that the number of capsules per day you have to take of your multivitamin changes your likelihood of falling pregnant. The more capsules (they studied up to 4) the better you do. I almost never prescribe multivitamins. They are a little bit of everything, and not a lot of anything. So maybe if we increase the number of capsules, we do better as far as the dose. Just a hunch. My preference is to use a multi that has activated folic acid (MTHF) instead of plain folic acid. In some provinces and states, drug plans will cover specific multivitamins that are made by pharmaceutical companies. To the best of my knowledge, most haven't adjusted their folic acid to reflect the most recent research. Pay out-of-pocket if you have to. It is worth it.

> Multivitamins are a little bit of everything, and not a lot of anything.

As a bit of a side-note, your multivitamin may protect you against some of the dietary indiscretions you have, such as alcohol. In one study women who used a multivitamin seemed to have less alcohol-associated miscarriage than women who did not use a multi[105]. I'm not suggesting your multi is a hall pass for booze. But it is interesting that a multi seems to improve other risk factors for miscarriage, even if they don't decrease miscarriage rates themselves.

YOU MIGHT NEED IRON (ESPECIALLY IF YOU ARE DEFICIENT)

We have got a bit of a gap with our recommendations for iron supplementation, and part of that is based on how we screen women with prenatal blood work. We are often testing your hemoglobin, not your actual iron storage, and the evidence suggests that in pregnancy, we should be dosing you based on your iron storage. One of those good old public-health-screening-not-actually-guiding-us-to-treating-you-best situations. My fave! Many women struggle to keep their iron storage up in their menstruating years. It is a bit of an uphill battle against monthly blood loss, especially if you have a low iron diet or if you have heavy periods. Most studies on iron have looked at premature labour rather than a miscarriage. But still, I'd recommend you get tested and treat your deficiency if you have one.

VITAMIN D

Most patients not only have a vitamin D deficiency but a practitioner deficiency. To adequately address low vitamin D, you need both a blood test and a practitioner who can prescribe it.

I am a big advocate for testing and treating vitamin D in all women looking to conceive. Vitamin D is one of the few supplements that has been well established to improve infant health outcomes in pregnancy, so even beyond the connection with miscarriage, we don't want our pregnant women to walk around with low levels of vitamin D.

Vitamin D and miscarriage is a curious topic. Most conditions that increase the risk of miscarriage such as Hashimoto's, APS and PCOS have a strong connection to vitamin D deficiency[22,87,106–108]. Women with these medical conditions are deficient more often than not, and we can see improvements in other symptoms and body systems (glucose, immune factors, antibodies) when we restore vitamin D levels to normal.

In one observational study, it was found that for every point increase of vitamin D women had on blood work, their overall risk of miscarriage went down by 1%[109]. The curious thing was, they did not look at specific medical conditions, but grouped all women into one pile. This is important

CHAPTER 7 — NUTRITIONAL SUPPLEMENTS

because we don't usually see these kinds of results if we put 'healthy' women in the same study group as women with medical conditions. Regardless of their baseline health, every single point saved them 1% risk. This is huge.

If you are considering IVF, there's evidence that being vitamin D replete improves your treatment success and increases live birth rate[110]. The one study that reviewed all the data did not find a reduction in miscarriage, but overall the women who had enough vitamin D had more babies. Sounds good to me.

Vitamin D is concentrated in the uterine lining, or "decidua" and plays a role in the immune system being accepting of the foreign body (baby) into the environment. Women with recurrent miscarriage have different vitamin D receptors than women without and may produce less vitamin D when exposed to sunlight than women who have never miscarried[111]. This concentration of vitamin D at the maternal-fetal interface (medicine-code for mom-baby connection) is likely a clue why deficiency is creating a problem. Vitamin D supplementation lowers the immune activity in women with recurrent miscarriage and APS and improves the uterine lining of women with PCOS. However, we have yet to see a good trial where we give women vitamin D, and they stop miscarrying.

Women with Hashimoto's can lower their TPO antibodies in only two ways, and vitamin D is one of them. One study had women use 1200-4000 IU for four months and decreased their TPO by about 20%[112]. The prescription was based on their lab work and dosed to maintain adequate blood levels. Another study on Vitamin D and TPO showed a 60% reduction with very heroic dosing for eight weeks[87]. If your thyroid is involved, get your sunshine vitamin tested.

When I graduated from school the lower limit of the vitamin D reference range was 60% lower than what it currently is. We have changed the healthy range a few times, as we learn the importance of this nutrient in overall health. I don't want to make this simple vitamin out to be total health panacea. I think there's way more to the story here. Low vitamin D may be a marker for something else that is highly correlated to your health: outdoor exercise. Maybe women who never go outside to exercise, miscarry more often, and have more autoimmune disease. It is possible. Either way, being deficient has too many health risks and sets you up for more complications in your pregnancy such as premature labour and gestational diabetes. Test. Treat. End of story, at least for now.

The challenge with dosing for miscarriage prevention is:

* Anything-over 1000 IU in many regions is considered a prescription, and
* we should dose you based on your lab work.

You can see my difficulty in writing this chapter! Really what you need is a practitioner who will first test you, and then prescribe based on your personal needs.

GENERAL RECOMMENDATIONS

Get tested before using higher dosing, but in the meantime use 1000 IU vitamin D per day. Anything higher may be considered a prescription where you live, and will require a qualified practitioner to give you the final okay.

VITAMIN C AND ANTIOXIDANTS

Across all of the women's health conditions I treat (menstrual cramps, PMS, fertility and menopause) there is a theme to the underlying dietary recommendations: we need more antioxidants. If we feed antioxidant vegetable powders to menopausal women their hot flashes resolve. If we give weak antioxidants to women with endometriosis or cramps their pain goes down[54,62,113]. If we feed women a few more fruits and veggies their PMS symptoms improve[114]. So it's not a huge stretch to see how the antioxidant class of nutrients could impact miscarriage too.

By incorporating more fruits and vegetables into one's diet, we see more micronutrients taken in (micronutrient deficiencies are a big cause of miscarriage in developing nations[115]), more fibre and more antioxidants. Antioxidants have been given as supplements in a few studies, but to date, we haven't really exhausted this subject in a way I'd like see. The most relevant study fed women with LPD (Luteal Phase Defect) 750 mg of Vitamin C as a supplement, and found that it protected the cells of their corpus luteum[43]. This boosted their progesterone production significantly. In this particular study they didn't see a huge difference in miscarriage rates, but for pennies spent on a harmless and possibly helpful supplement, I'd suggest everyone could use more vitamin C in their life. Be sure you get at least 1000 mg. A few bioflavonoids are considered contraindicated in pregnancy such as Quercetin, so avoid any Vitamin C supplements that have a bunch of other ingredients in them. You don't need them.

As a side note, if you have a guinea pig that can't get pregnant, you should feed her vitamin C. Vitamin C deficiency is a major cause of infertility in guinea pigs apparently.

MELATONIN

Melatonin is traditionally thought of as a sleep hormone, and that is not wrong. But that title certainly underestimates the importance of this hormone in overall health and miscarriage risk.

You already produce melatonin naturally, in a daily pattern, with levels increasing in the evening to help initiate sleep. It is produced from a tiny gland in the brain in response to lowered daylight, and it supports many biological functions such as sleep and reproduction. Reproduction in most species is seasonal, with melatonin having a role in either promoting or suppressing fertility. Animals reproduce at different times of the year depending on how long they are pregnant, and when resources are most available based on the season (they don't want to have a baby in the middle of winter!). Funnily a lot of the research on melatonin is in

CHAPTER 7 — NUTRITIONAL SUPPLEMENTS

farm animals, where we want them to have babies all year long, against their natural yearly cycle.

When we look at miscarriage in general, women who work night shift have an increased risk of miscarriage, even if they are pretty healthy otherwise[116]. Melatonin levels are lower in women who work night shift, but their other hormones (LH and FSH) are the same as their daytime-working sisters. Meaning that melatonin is independently having an impact on fertility, regardless of how good the rest of your hormones look. This also points to some significant problems for shift workers. Low melatonin levels have also been linked to pain, inflammation and the immune system in shift workers. Being awake at night reduces your natural production of melatonin — since in addition to not sleeping, you are exposed to artificial light — and this prevents women from gaining the antioxidant benefits of this hormone, putting them at risk of severe diseases such as breast cancer (a topic for another book).

Working night shift wreaks havoc on your cycle length too. Women who work the night shift for two years are more likely to have short or long cycles (less than 21 days or more than 40 days)[117]. There is likely more to this story, but you can see the problem. Working when you are supposed to be sleeping is not good for your fertility.

If you are a night shift worker, I'm guessing quitting your job is not a viable answer. My suggestion is to check for other unhealthy habits that have crept in during your night shift work that may be some contributing in part to your health and fertility issues. We know that women who work the night shift are less active and are more overweight than women who don't. Don't let this be part of your picture. Step away from the donuts girl!

There is also evidence that swapping between days and nights may eliminate some of the detriment of straight night shifts. *Maybe put in for a shift change?* In one study that followed almost 90,000 women who miscarried, avoiding night shift was one of their penultimate recommendations[116]. I cannot say it enough.

Because it is an antioxidant, Melatonin improves oxidative-stress, which is the fancy title for dysfunction that happens as a result of an imbalance between levels of oxidation and antioxidants. Our bodies create oxidants as part of regular wear and tear, and we are exposed to them in the environment. If you don't eat enough antioxidants, or cannot produce them fast enough, this imbalance can lead to inflammation, cell destruction and immune system dysfunction. Inflammation, cell destruction and immune dysfunction has shown up in almost every syndrome related to miscarriage so far.

Melatonin has mostly been researched for improving egg health and quality in IVF. We are even growing eggs in gels containing melatonin in IVF cycles and having better outcomes[118,119] Now isn't this interesting! If we take an egg out and expose it to melatonin, the egg is healthier, and the cycle is more effective. IVF eggs are particularly at risk for oxidative stress. They are taken out of their cosy follicular fluid environment and exposed to more oxygen and handling than eggs developed in their natural environment.

Critics of my melatonin suggestion may say that the melatonin works in IVF because we created the problem with the solution (we created oxidative stress by doing IVF) and it is not going to be the same in non-IVF cycles. To defend my point, melatonin receptors are in the ovary, it concentrates in the pelvis during the luteal phase, and we can measure the oxidative breakdown of eggs in all women, sometimes starting as soon as 8 hours after ovulation.

Most conditions that increase the risk of miscarriage have elevated oxidative stress. I don't think it is a huge leap based on all of this that melatonin may reduce miscarriage. *Are you with me?*

Where we have the best evidence is using melatonin in women with luteal phase defect. Melatonin increases luteal phase progesterone levels and reduced risk of miscarriage in women with diagnosed LPD[45,120]. In these studies, women were supplemented 3 mg of melatonin at bedtime for the month before their insemination at a fertility clinic. Melatonin protects your progesterone-producing cells from being harmed (which we think is part of the problem in LPD) and keeps them pumping out progesterone longer. There are actually over 400 articles on the connection between progesterone and melatonin, but 300 of them are in farm animals. Melatonin is standard care for treating infertility in farm animals. I wonder who the genius was that decided to try it in humans?

Regardless of the cause of infertility or miscarriage, melatonin given to women undergoing IVF cycles improves egg quality and increases the likelihood of a successful cycle[47]. Even taken as little as from day 1-5 of the cycle is having positive outcomes on birth rates in all women in fertility clinics so maybe this is something we should consider for all women, not just women with low progesterone and LPD.

Melatonin has been shown to reduce the need for pain medication in women with endometriosis, by reducing inflammation[55], and improves hormone release in women with premature ovarian failure due to its antioxidant effect[121]. It has been combined with other treatments for women with PCOS undergoing IVF[122], and as I mentioned earlier, it is growing healthier eggs when we add it to growth mediums in IVF. My guess is that we will see many more studies connecting melatonin to miscarriage in the next few years with positive results.

There are ways you can improve your melatonin levels naturally such as reducing light exposure between 6 pm, and 7 am and avoiding caffeine and alcohol since both lower melatonin production. Some mood medications lower melatonin, but that should be discussed with your doctor. There are natural sources of melatonin, such as dark tart cherry juice, but read me loud and clear that we have no evidence that cherry juice reduces miscarriage.

Taking melatonin as a supplement does not interfere with your ability to make your own. This is a prevalent myth I bust when prescribing it. Melatonin is out of your system fast (for some women with insomnia it may not even last the full night sleep, and you will still wake up in the early morning). Taking it every night does not change your production, but does change the peak amount in your blood. It should be taken nightly at the same time, not just when you know you're in for bad sleep. Technically melatonin improves mood and energy even if you don't sleep more. Kind of cool if you ask me.

There is a threshold for taking too much for hormone function, with high doses of melatonin possibly suppressing ovulation in women who are also taking progesterone (which should be almost all of you). Three milligrams appear to be the most studied dose, and as I said, even if it does not knock you out, it is still exerting positive effects on hormones and fertility.

GENERAL RECOMMENDATIONS

* 3 mg melatonin nightly for at least 1-2 months before conception for luteal phase defect.
* Also, consider as part of a total fertility plan for women with premature ovarian failure, endometriosis or PCOS.

FISH OIL

Omega-3 fats found in fish have an anti-inflammatory effect in the body, especially in the uterus. Omega-3s have been well studied for menstrual cramps, and they work by incorporating themselves into a cell structure, and decreasing inflammation when those cells are shed with each cycle.

Women who are overweight at the time of their IVF cycle have better success rates if they use omega-3 oils throughout their fertility care[123] and even having just one discussion about healthy eating habits prior to conception improves a woman's fish intake[124].

When it comes specifically to miscarriage, the goal of using omega-3 fats is to improve uterine blood flow, reduce inflammation and decrease any clotting problems, especially if you have been diagnosed with antiphospholipid syndrome. Using higher doses of fish oil has been shown to improve uterine blood flow in women with any cause of recurrent miscarriage[125]. Unfortunately, they did not report birth rate; they just scanned them with an ultrasound looking at blood flow. Fish oil has been compared with Aspirin for reducing miscarriage in women with APS, or unexplained recurrent miscarriage — that we would otherwise treat with anti-coagulant drugs[92].

Only population data has looked at the use of plant-based omega-3s, and we have no evidence to use flax, hemp or chia-based oils for clotting disorders or improving uterine blood flow. Of course, healthy fats from veggie sources are helpful, but if you are a recurrent miscarrier, they may not be strong enough to get the effect you need. Very little plant-based omega-3 is turned into the 'active' ingredient you need to have the best outcome.

GENERAL RECOMMENDATIONS

* If you have been diagnosed with APS, or "unexplained recurrent miscarriage" use fish oil containing EPA and DHA with a total fish oil dose of 4 grams per day. (the EPA and DHA dose will be less than this, but it is important to choose a product that delivers high amounts of EPA and DHA per capsule)
* If you are overweight and are exploring fertility care, fish oil capsules and dietary omega-3s from vegetarian sources should be included in your diet.
* All women should incorporate more fish into their diet eating 2-3 servings per week.

SELENIUM

Selenium is a mineral that is found in soil, nuts and seeds. It is an integral part of optimal thyroid function, and at a population level, is found to be lower in groups who test positive for autoimmune thyroiditis (Hashimoto's). As a treatment, selenium has been shown to lower thyroid antibodies enough to consider it a mainstay of treatment for women with Hashimoto's Thyroiditis (HT)[85,86,88,126,127].

The type of selenium seems to matter, with selenomethionine being the most absorbable form. Some studies that have found no effect when using selenium with HT, and review articles that haven't distinguished between different selenium salts will conclude that overall selenium does not affect thyroid antibodies. If we only look at the studies on selenomethionine, there is an effect, but it takes 3-6 months to see it.

Selenium has been studied outside of the world of fertility to restore thyroid function in HT with and without medication. In the fertility world, I always suggest pairing selenium with medication to get us to our endpoint. It is what the research suggests, and likely will achieve the ultimate baby-goal faster and more often than using the supplement alone.

Dietary selenium is also essential for women trying to conceive, and a connection has been made between selenium and luteal phase defect likely through the healthy foods that include selenium[128]. For every ten micrograms of selenium eaten as part of their diet, there was a significant reduction in the risk of having a luteal phase defect. The study was looking at the Mediterranean diet, and of course, selenium is found in nuts. So, we can probably safely say that the healthier the diet is, and the more nuts and seeds incorporated, the more likely women are to ovulate and ovulate well.

There is a dark side of selenium in the world of blood sugar regulation, with many studies on diabetic patients showing a worsening of insulin resistance when selenium is supplemented. A couple of studies have shown the same problem in women with PCOS[129,130].

So now what? Here are my recommendations:

* If you have POCS and you don't have HT, you don't need selenium.

- ✱ If you have HT, you need selenium.
- ✱ If you have both? Well, shoot.

Speak with your practitioner about what your biggest obstacle is or see if any of the other TPO lowering strategies (Vitamin D) or insulin-regulating strategies could potentially negate the situation. I haven't found research on it, so I cannot make a generalized conclusion for you.

Once you get pregnant, you likely should continue some selenium supplementation. Studies are using as low as 60-200 mcg on-going in pregnancy, and although your antibodies may fluctuate up or down, the selenium still supports thyroid function in women who have tested positive for TPO before getting pregnant. Your multivitamin may be enough. Check the label.

GENERAL RECOMMENDATIONS

- ✱ 200 micrograms of selenomethionine in women who have tested positive for anti-thyroid antibodies (TPO or Anti-TG).
- ✱ Avoid additional selenium use above what is in a multivitamin in women with PCOS, insulin resistance, type 2 diabetes or who do not have low thyroid but are overweight and attempting to get pregnant.

NAC

N-Acetyl-Cysteine (NAC) is an antioxidant-like amino acid (protein building block) that has some unique characteristics that make it much more exciting than her other amino-acid sisters in the world of fertility.

NAC has been studied mostly in PCOS to improve insulin resistance and ovulation rates, and when we pool all of the studies together, we find that women with PCOS who take NAC ovulate more, have 3 times more live births, and it even supports women who have already tried clomiphene and who have failed[131]. (To the tune of 5x more successful in their next fertility round.)

This is likely owed to the impact NAC has on insulin and blood sugar. Because it has a similar action to Metformin, the diabetes drug commonly prescribed for PCOS, most research compares NAC to Metformin, and generally, Metformin wins in the head to head comparison. We know Metformin carries with it a lot of gastro-side effects, and in women who cannot tolerate it, NAC becomes a good choice. What we don't know is what happens if we use them together.

When it comes to miscarriage, we can see improved live birth rates, but only one study has looked at miscarriage specifically[132]. The study used NAC a few days a month (Day 3-7) for a year in women who had just had ovarian drilling. I think I used to cringe at the name "ovarian drilling" just based on the visual, but in reality, this fertility-saving treatment for some women can be the difference maker, especially if we suspect high androgens (testosterone) being the major culprit for the lack of fertility.

The "drilling" is a removal of some ovarian tissue, which in women with PCOS, are overproducing the wrong hormones at the wrong times. Taking out some of the tissue that is overproducing testosterone can allow the stunted eggs to develop and it increases ovulation and pregnancy rates. The research suggests that transvaginal ovarian drilling reduces your risk of scaring, and improves fertility, so be sure to talk to your fertility clinic about which procedure they use.

Adding NAC to the mix for the year following the procedure results in higher ovulation rates, higher pregnancy rates, higher live birth rates and a much lower miscarriage rate. In the specific study, the miscarriage rate went from 23% in the placebo group to 8% in the treated group. That's comparable to the general population. Not bad for a supplement taken five days a month.

I don't often use NAC in other fertility concerns, reserving it only for my PCOS ladies. We don't have the evidence to use it anywhere else. Yes, it is an amazing nutrient, but not everyone seems to need it. Ask me again in 5 years, and maybe we will know more.

GENERAL RECOMMENDATIONS FOR NAC

* 1200 mg per day (divided up through the day) from day 3-7 (5 days total) in women who have had previous ovarian drilling.

* 1200 mg per day every day for women with PCOS who are not ovulating often, and who have elevated fasting insulin or who have a previously failed clomiphene cycle and are going to try again.

BERBERINE

Berberine is another condition-specific herb (PCOS ladies, listen up) that has a role in improving the success of IVF, and reduces miscarriage even better than some of the standard drugs. And you have likely never heard of it. Berberine is an active ingredient in a bunch of herbs, with traditional uses as an antibiotic, it has been well used for upper respiratory tract infections and acne to wipe out the bacteria involved.

In the fertility world, we have started to recognize the use of Berberine to support women with PCOS, because in addition to it is pathogen-killing properties, it works in the same mechanism as Metformin to reduce blood sugar and insulin—very cool if you ask me.

In most other fields such as cancer or diabetes, I'm not likely to recommend Berberine over Metformin. Metformin is safe and is generally thought of as the more effective drug of the two when compared head to head. But in the world of miscarriage, we have some evidence that Berberine may do a slightly better job[29].

Both Metformin and Berberine lower androgens and insulin. They both improve ovulation rates and pregnancy rates in women with PCOS. However, when compared to Metformin, Berberine has a more well-rounded treatment effect in women with PCOS (meaning it improves more blood work markers—mostly cardiovascular) and has a higher live birth rate and lower miscarriage rate than Metformin, with a way fewer side effects.

The cool part about the study is that these warrior women in the Berberine study had already been trying to conceive for two years. Two years! When we watch a treatment help our least likely group of women to get pregnant, get pregnant, then we are probably on to something big.

If you have been offered Metformin by your fertility doctor, great! Stick with it, slap on some probiotics to eliminate the GI side effects and you're off to the races. If you are not being actively treated for high insulin, and have PCOS, and are thinking about IVF or some other protocol, then I'd get on Berberine until you are offered medication. If you want to quit your Metformin because of the side effects (Metformin is very safe in pregnancy by the way, and I recommend for patients to discuss this option with their doctors often), then you have got an alternative. It all depends on what your goals are.

GENERAL RECOMMENDATIONS FOR BERBERINE

- One capsule (500 mg) three times per day with a meal for women with PCOS who are not actively being treated with medication for blood sugar and insulin, or for women who cannot tolerate standard care (Metformin) due to side effects.

FOLIC ACID

When I was a student, "active folate" was a new thing. Since you know I did not go to school with the dinosaurs; you can tell that this idea of genes, methylation defects, and that every woman is different, is pretty new. I looked at Methyltetrahydrofolate (herein referred to as MTHF or "active folate") and compared it to folic acid. I was utterly oblivious to the gene issues with folic acid (as was much of the world) and thought the only benefit to active folate was how quickly it raises folic acid levels in the blood.

I wasn't wrong. MTHF increases folic acid levels way faster than folate, which can take up to 12-24 weeks when taken as part of a regular prenatal to adequately protect your baby from a neural tube defect. Now for our Type-A mamas-to-be, you may be planning your next 24 weeks beautifully and have started your prenatal in time. But for us fly-by-the-seat-of-our-booty-shorts Type-B ladies (I'm Type B and proud), we realized we wanted to get pregnant (or that we already were pregnant) with no forward thought whatsoever. Using high dose MTHF can raise folate levels in about two weeks. High enough to prevent neural tube defects and the other pressing concerns that are associated with low folic acid levels. If you smoke, well your second step is to get on high dose MTHF (first is to initiate a quit-plan). Smoking makes raising your folate levels harder. So, you will need more than the average Jane[133].

I'm not going to cover the public-health concepts about folic acid. That's likely been beaten into you by now. Folic acid reduces a lot of things that can go wrong in fetal development.

When it comes to miscarriage, it is likely the link with homocysteine that makes folic acid so important. You see, MTHF (not folate) is required to lower homocysteine. We know that homocysteine causes miscarriage. So why would the government recommend folate if it is not the thing that we're after? Genetics my dear. Genetics.

Some women can take plain old folic acid and turn it into MTHF brilliantly. All by herself. No help. So, give her some folate, and she will lower her homocysteine and likely never miscarry and have as many babies as her heart desires. Some women on the other hand, cannot. Feed them all the folate you want, and they cannot make MTHF. Oops. Now we have a problem. If all dietary folate cannot be used to lower homocysteine, then what happens?

Likely a miscarriage, that's what.

At this moment in time, testing for MTHF for recurrent pregnancy loss does not help us any more than just taking active folate[26]. It has been well looked at, and just taking high dose MTHF (not smoking) and monitoring homocysteine is the best way to go[75]. Don't spend the money on the test, or waste time waiting for the results. There are practitioners who will disagree with me, but remember, I'm just talking miscarriage. Perhaps there are scenarios where testing makes sense. For miscarriage, it does not. Have I flogged that horse enough?

Our public health dosing for folic acid over the years has been a bit of a drama if you ask me, and a great reflection of how we tend to treat things conventionally in general. We used to recommend 400 micrograms of folate (plain old folate) unless you had already had a neural tube defect, and then you get 5,000 micrograms (5 mg).

Yep, you read that right. We waited until you had a problem, then we gave you more of the harmless nutrient that some of you can't metabolize efficiently. Throw me a bone! The other problem is that here in many parts of Canada, folic acid over 1 mg is considered a prescription. Why? No idea. I looked into it, and all I could find is the list of who needs high dose folate. Interestingly Health Canada lists the times when high dose folate should be considered.

PUBLIC HEALTH VERSION: When to consider high dose folic acid supplementation

- Poor dietary habits
- Chronic dieting or low carbohydrate diets (avoiding the fortified flour)
- Low income
- Using rice as a staple in the diet or other non-fortified foods
- Personal or family history of neural tube defects or other congenital disorders
- Medications that interfere with folate metabolism
- Alcohol use/abuse

- ✱ Poor absorption in the digestive system or a disease of the digestive system (including gastric bypass)
- ✱ Liver disease
- ✱ Kidney dialysis
- ✱ Obesity
- ✱ Diabetes
- ✱ Impaired glucose metabolism
- ✱ Hyperinsulinemia (high insulin in the blood)

Well? What do you think of the list?

How many of you fall into the public health list of ladies who need high dose folate? If you have PCOS, have miscarried before, are overweight, drink at all, smoke (they forgot that one apparently), or are on a gluten-free diet, or-or-or... etc. You get the picture. It is all of you.

So, let's try that again.

JORDAN'S VERSION: when to consider high dose folic acid supplementation

Everyone.

Diet is not an excellent source of folate for the prevention of miscarriage and neural tube defects. It is in veggies, and in fortified flour, but we still find that if women supplement they do better. Interestingly there is a component in green tea that may block the activation of folate from inactive to MTHF. Maybe it is a bit of an over-kill recommendation, but there is some loose science on the subject. So, if you're not a big green tea drinker, don't start.

GENERAL RECOMMENDATIONS

* No, I cannot recommend taking more than 1 mg of active folate given that it is a prescription. So, here's what I would suggest. Take a good quality multivitamin with MTHF as the source of folate, and at least 1 milligram per day. Don't do things that get in the way of folate metabolism (smoke, drink, excessive green tea) and find a practitioner who is willing to prescribe MTHF in a dose of 4-5 mg per day.

VITAMIN B12

My opinion around B12 is similar to vitamin D. Test and treat. If you are deficient, that's bad. Just treat it. There are a few studies that have looked at the risk of miscarriage with B12 deficiency, and have found a correlation. They are in developing nations, so maybe not as applicable to our North American sisters. That said, in the largest of the studies on the topic, they used the same deficiency cut off that we use here (>200 pg/ml) so if it's been flagged on your blood work, it doesn't matter where you live, you should treat it[134].

Generally B12 levels respond really well to oral supplementation, and practitioners can often pick out who is supplementing just by looking at your lab work. Most multi-vitamins will contain about 400 mcg, which may be enough to pull you out of the basement of deficiency. Maybe take a bit more. You don't necessarily need injections—as most of the data suggests that a B12 supplement will raise you levels just as well as an injection. If you like being injected, then by all means!

GENERAL RECOMMENDATIONS

Have your B12 levels tested and treat it if you are frankly deficient and flagged on your lab work. Take at least 400 mcg per day to lower homocysteine, and keep your levels sufficient. If you are vegan or vegetarian, you may require higher levels given that your diet is low. 1000-5000 mcg is generally safe, and may improve other parts of your health such as fatigue and mood. There are multiple forms of B12, and although none of them have been studied specifically for miscarriage, I generally suggest the methylated version (methylcobalamin) for the methylation support in the homocysteine pathways.

HORMONES

The use of hormones for miscarriage support has been well studied, with over 75% of fertility clinics in North America now on board to use progesterone as support after IVF and IUI[7]. I remember when I got pregnant the fourth time *(remember I had three miscarriages),* I asked my family doctor for a prescription for progesterone. He wasn't on board but did it anyway. You should not have to beg for hormonal support. The evidence is clear — even if we don't know why you miscarry, ("unexplained miscarriage") progesterone support is going to help you[50].

As for the other hormones, unfortunately, we don't have a great way of testing or treating hormone deficiencies in early pregnancy. We know they are there, but we are not sure what to do about it. An excellent study looked at blood levels of women with a threatened miscarriage who were bleeding before 28 weeks, and compared it to healthy women who were not spotting. Most hormones (Estrogen, testosterone, DHEA) were lower in the women who had threatened miscarriage compared to the women who were not spotting[135]. So, we know there is a connection, but we don't know how to support you. This section will present on what we know to date on using hormones to prevent miscarriage.

DHEA FOR PREMATURE OVARIAN FAILURE

DHEA has been studied mostly in women with premature ovarian failure (POF). POF, even once we overcome the ovarian issues and have successful egg retrieval, it still leaves women at risk of miscarriage. DHEA not only improves the quality of the eggs retrieved but also decreases the risk of miscarriage once women undergo their IVF cycle[136]. The dose of DHEA needed to work borders on side effects (I haven't seen a woman who did not have side effects) with about 75-90 mg per day required for the result. One study showed that they could reduce the miscarriage rate of POF women down to a normal IVF population by using DHEA, which is encouraging, but we need to see a bit more on this topic to say without a shadow of a doubt it helps. Truthfully if you have POF and are scheduled for an IVF, you should talk to your doctor about DHEA anyways. It helps improve oocyte maturity, and the number of follicles retrieved and live birth rate. Again, dose bordering on side effects, and there is not much we can do except wait for the bloated-acne-laden four months out.

ESTROGEN, TESTOSTERONE, AND OTHERS.

Although other hormones are related to fertility in general, and some of you may have experienced some add-back therapy of estrogen for thin uterine lining, hot flashes during lengthy down-regulation protocols or for other deficiencies, there is no data to date they help with miscarriage. Moving on to the big show: progesterone.

PROGESTERONE (EVERYONE NEEDS TO READ THIS PART)

After your beautiful egg has been released, and before that baby-to-be implants and starts creating his or her hormones, they rely on you to produce enough progesterone to maintain the pregnancy. This combined with the fact that most risk factors for infertility and miscarriage are related to reduced progesterone levels is why there is a need for progesterone supplementation in women at risk. This is also why you should not have to beat your practitioner over the head for a prescription. You need it.

As you read earlier, most causes of miscarriage are linked to issues with progesterone production (PCOS, POF, LPD, Endometriosis) or have a reduced "sensitivity" to the progesterone you do make (LPD, Endometriosis). During that critical window after fertilization and before stable implantation, the uterus is supposed to be flooded with progesterone. This establishes blood flow and keeps the pregnancy viable. We can mimic this with bio-identical progesterone made into vaginal suppositories and help reduce miscarriage rates in almost all women.

Progesterone can be given in multiple ways (orally, injection or in cream), but the vaginal suppository route is the most effective[137]. It should be started right after your IVF procedure, right after your IUI, or right after ovulation. The studies have looked at using it as few as five days, or as long as six weeks in most cases, with a few rarer studies using it up to 28 weeks[50]. The suppositories are messy, but when compared with the other routes of administration, it works much better. Worth the mess, invest in some panty liners.

Now, of course, using a drug is not without risk. We have seen slightly increased risks of gestational diabetes (GD) and large for gestational age babies in women who have used progesterone[31]. This would show up in your week-16 oral glucose tolerance test (drink the drink, wait and be tested). Women who have used progesterone have an increased risk of high fasting glucose and high glucose after the drink. This increases the risk for gestational diabetes. What we don't know yet is if women who need progesterone are at more significant risk for GD anyways, so maybe the drug is just a random association because we use it in women already at risk, but time will tell. This is why I generally use it for six weeks or less.

Also, if you have a history of cervical dysplasia, progesterone use has been associated with more progression of dysplasia, and a greater need for the use of surgical techniques when women had used progesterone vaginally[138]. The study on dysplasia was trying to look at using progesterone to TREAT cervical dysplasia, and instead, it worsened it. They don't know why and neither do I.

I would treat your dysplasia before you get pregnant anyway, so maybe that solves this problem. To recap, you all likely need progesterone. Please work with someone well versed enough in this field to help you. Before Naturopathic Doctors had prescribing rights in Ontario, I sent many letters to doctors to advocate for my women. Now I can support them entirely, so I encourage you to connect with someone who can too.

GENERAL RECOMMENDATIONS FOR HORMONES

* DHEA 25 mg three times per day for four months before IVF cycle in women with premature ovarian failure.

* Progesterone 100-200 mg twice per day in vaginal suppository starting from ovulation, IVF or IUI procedure until 4-6 weeks gestation, or until HCG testing or ultrasound confirms a viable pregnancy.

CHAPTER 8

YOU. CAN. DO. THIS.

We have a problem in medicine—and you're being swept along with it. Realistically, we know the root of many diseases are linked to diet and lifestyle—but we assume that patients are not interested, cannot or will not do the work to make an impact on their health.

Personally, I haven't met a more motivated group of women—then those who understand that their actions will make a difference to their reproductive health. Whether it is miscarriage, PMS, menopause, migraines or breast cancer, women who think they can impact their health, do just that.

Medicine has done a massive disservice to the public by gate keeping instead of collaborating—resulting in many patients feeling victimized by their situation. That they are at the mercy of their hormones or worse still, that they are not "destined" to have children.

Though I say a lot in this book about what you should be doing, I hope you can see my efforts to empower you through this process. I am in no way suggesting that your last miscarriage was your fault—or if you have another one that it is your fault. What I'm suggesting is that if you make changes towards a healthier lifestyle and advocate for yourself—it will be *your work* that caused you not to miscarry. My hope is that, we medical professionals do a better job of supporting patients through this process.

Well, sister put on your heels, or runners, or flip-flops and start changing things for yourself. It's not going to be easy, but won't it all be worth it, if you carry to term?

You did it!

Your journey starts now. We have goals of reaching thousands of women, and you can also have an impact on another woman's life and help her get started on her own fertility journey.

Our reach depends on our readers sharing their story and by leaving an Amazon review. Your experience reading the book matters to us and can help other women and couples if you leave a review on the Amazon website.

Thank you for contributing to our greater mission of reducing stigma around miscarriage and improving access to care for couples who experience miscarriage and pregnancy loss.

xoxo Jordan.

AFTERWORD
FOR THE SWIMMERS

I'm going to make a lateral move away from just talking about miscarriage in these final pages, to talk a bit about male infertility in general. We don't have the depth of research I would like to see on how sperm health impacts miscarriage rates. I will explain why in a second, but I want to be clear. Miscarriages are different than other causes of infertility. You already know this. You can get pregnant, but you cannot stay pregnant. We have laser focused on it all along through the book. We haven't been wishy-washy about how to be a one-with-the-universe healthy goddess to conceive. Yes, I want you healthy, but mostly I want you not to miscarry.

We cannot ignore the men — but so far, the research has. We have very few actual studies on miscarriages as it relates to sperm health. But it felt like if I did not include some information on how to have healthier sperm, I was making it all about you. It's not. It just can't be. You know it, and I know it.

So here we are, talking a bit about fertility in general as it pertains to your male counterpart.

Male infertility is potentially easier to treat than female infertility if we could get their freaking butts in the doctor's office. Study after study has shown that we generally don't assess males—up to a quarter of infertile couples never have the male partner evaluated at all, and because of the advances in technology in reproductive medicine, we have for the most part taken the male's health out of the equation. This has had a downstream effect in the research because instead of investigating why the male may be struggling with low counts, poor sperm quality or other causes of infertility we check the box that says "male infertility" on his chart and then use technology to jump over the problem. Only recently have I started to see some focus on studies correlating total sperm quality and quantity with IVF success rates. Again, in the past, we just selected the couple sperm that looked the healthiest and washed the situation of the rest, but even if we choose a man's best swimmer, if he had low counts to begin with, you have a higher likelihood of IVF failure.

Sperm is made on the daily, which had led us to believe that perhaps a man's health history does not have as great of an impact on his sperm as a woman's history has on her eggs (which are with her for her entire life). Unfortunately, and not surprisingly, we were not even close to being right. Even a woman's health during pregnancy can have an impact on her future son's sperm quality, and so even if a male partner has cleaned up his act from his teens and 20's, he may still have residual changes to his fertility from bad behaviors in his past. Don't fret; there are solutions. I want you to recognize that 1) your dude needs to be tested, and 2) his total health matters as much as yours.

AFTERWORD — FOR THE SWIMMERS

There are a lot of reasons why a man's sperm could be affected over his lifetime, and there are some great checklists to look at when trying to decide if your male partner is at risk of low fertility. The physical causes include things like previous trauma or surgeries (including surgery for undescended testicles when he was a baby), varicose veins of the scrotum, or past infections such as mumps, testicular infections, chemotherapy exposure or other medications that lower sperm health.

As a Naturopathic Doctor, I often end up focusing a lot on the endocrine and metabolic causes of low sperm. This is partly because no other practitioners focus on it, and partly because that's where I can have the most significant impact. However, it is essential that you don't ignore the other possible contributors. Your male partner needs his medications assessed to see if he's taking something that could be getting in the way and should have a good health history and physical exam done with an experienced practitioner.

Laboratory assessment for male infertility should include a hormone panel looking at pituitary hormones such as FSH and LH and testicular hormones such as testosterone. Estrogen is a valuable hormone to assess given the impact of weight and BMI on male hormone levels, but in the medical community, they only add this test if the male has abnormal breast tissue development. I'd advocate having the test is done, as well as SHBG, the protein in the blood that carries sex hormones. Testosterone to Estrogen ratios is a new measure of metabolic health and wellness in men.

As weight goes up, Estrogen goes up, and Testosterone goes down. We are finding that men with an altered T/E ratio have less sperm and have a harder time conceiving than men with better hormone balance. Insulin and glucose should also be tested, as well as prolactin (if he has erectile dysfunction) and cortisol. It is not a long list, but as I said, we often don't test the men at all.

LABORATORY ASSESSMENTS FOR MALE INFERTILITY

- LH and FSH to determine if testicular failure (they are high if the testicles are not responding)
- All measures of testosterone (total, free, bioavailable and DHT (dihydroxytestosterone))
- Estradiol: especially if overweight
- SHBG: especially if overweight
- Fasting Insulin and Glucose
- Prolactin: if erectile dysfunction is also present
- Cortisol
- Homocysteine, B12 and Folate

MEDICATIONS THAT IMPACT SPERM HEALTH

Some very common medications impact both sperm quality and quantity. One group studied the FDA approved medications that effect sperm quality[139], and some of our most commonly prescribed medications make the list. There are quite a few drugs on the list, so your man should have his medication list checked with his doctor. Some of the conventional drugs include corticosteroids (like inhalers), cardiovascular drugs and drugs to support mental health.

Antidepressants cause ejaculation latency (and is often used to treat premature ejaculation). Although these drugs don't seem to impact hormone levels, the infrequent ejaculation that comes with lower libido increases DNA damage in sperm[140].

Medications to control stomach acid have been shown to increase the risk of low sperm count in a few population-based studies. One research group connected it to homocysteine and folate levels, so if your male partner is on an acid suppressant, we may want to advocate for some testing of both folate and homocysteine to see if his medication is affecting his sperm quality[141].

Acetaminophen may decrease time to conception in couples and increases DNA damage in sperm. The higher Tylenol found in the male's urine, longer it takes a couple to conceive and the more significant the DNA damage in his sperm. We don't know yet if infrequent use causes the same problem, but in animal studies, even a single dose can affect sperm and might suppress production for up to 10 days after[142].

DIET FOR BETTER SPERM HEALTH

The most important part about diet and fertility for men is the impact that food has on weight. Men who weigh more than their ideal body weight have lower fertility. It influences all corners of fertility health and has a greater impact on Testosterone than age![143]. Excess weight carrying even causes increased testicular temperature from extra weight carried around the middle[144]. We cannot ignore the importance of weight loss in our overweight dads-to-be. Whatever strategy works for him is what we should use. Studies show that even men who are morbidly obese can have a return of their testicular function if they have dramatic weight loss[145]. There's hope. I'm a big advocate of choosing a weight loss plan that keeps patients happy and full. It does not have to be crazy-restrictive, or super-hard. It needs to invoke modest weight loss. If he cannot do it alone, he needs to enlist some help.

FOODS TO INCLUDE

An extensive study that pooled together research from 35 studies looking at male fertility found that the general dietary principles that improve sperm health are neither surprising or novel[146]. The Mediterranean-style diet we encourage for women is the same nutritional pattern that enhances fertility in men. High antioxidant/nutrient dense fruits and vegetables, high fish, nuts and monounsaturated fats all improved markers of male fertility.

AFTERWORD — FOR THE SWIMMERS

Because we haven't spent a lot of time on this topic in real live men (mostly animal or test tube data), I will cautiously recommend including the following healthy foods into the male diet. The foods have either been shown to have components that support better sperm quality or have been used to protect sperm undergoing freezing, thawing or insemination procedures. Not the kind of science I want to practice, but none of these are harmful, and if they kinda-sort of help, then let's do it.

Tomato juice, which is rich in the nutrient lycopene, has been shown to improve semen motility, even better than supplemented antioxidants[147]. I would not choose a pre-bottled-high-sodium tomato juice. I think using tomato paste, and tomato sauce liberally in the diet would have a similar effect. Both Green tea[148] and pomegranate[149] have been used to support antioxidant capacity in sperm that was being subject to harsh laboratory conditions. Drinking a ½ cup of pomegranate juice per day has a lot of health benefits in men anyway, so I'm happy to include this as part of a fertility diet. Green tea or matcha powder would also be an excellent addition for added antioxidant effects.

I also generally recommend beet juice and pistachios for male cardiovascular health especially if they have erectile dysfunction. The dose for pistachios to help is hefty (1/2 cup per day in one study) so include them in context with all of the other foods eaten in a day[150]. Be sure to incorporate lots of fruits and vegetables into your diet too. Even as low as a few hundred milligrams of vitamin C per day improves sperm quality[151,152].

The choice of fats in your male partner's diet may also have an impact on sperm health and quality. We have seen the benefits of olive oil, omega-3s and nuts a few times, and some more recent research is suggesting that the MCTs found in coconut oil may support better sperm quality as well[153].

FOODS TO AVOID

Ah, everyone's favorite topic. Foods that we love that are also terrible for us. I always like to keep this list as short and sweet as possible. If I cannot convince the patient as to why they need to eliminate foods, they won't. So I will keep it simple.

ALCOHOL

That's pretty much it boys. Cut the booze. Truthfully, we haven't bothered to study anything else. There are other bad behaviors in our diet that lower fertility (trans fats, simple sugars, processed or overcooked meats), but to date, the only real enemy your sperm have is alcohol. And there's no such thing as a 'safe amount'. The same study that looked at alcohol and failed IVF cycles in women tracked the alcohol intake for their male partners as well. IVF cycles failed twice as often when the men drank in the 4-week window before their transfer and the group that drank miscarried 2.7 times more often. The effect was dose-dependent, meaning that even one drink technically increased risk, and the more they had, the worse it was.

CAFFEINE

Caffeine intake in male partners has been shown to worsen the outcome of IVF or ISCI cycles, which is about as close as we can get to concrete data. Couples in the highest caffeine intake (which was only 250 mg of caffeine per day) had a live birth rate of 36% lower than males with the lowest caffeine intake[154].

GENERAL FOODS TO AVOID

That same study that showed benefits with the Mediterranean diet pattern also showed that diets high in full-fat dairy, soy, potatoes, and sugar-sweetened beverages all showed lower markers of male fertility such as sperm count. When they looked at actual birth rates, coffee, alcohol and processed meats were without a doubt linked to fewer babies.

Of interest, there has been a weak link between diets high in selenium and lower sperm measures, which would lead me to suggest that men shouldn't go out of their way to consume high levels of selenium, such as what would be found in a supplement. One study looked at dietary selenium, but they fed the men a considerable amount of this one nutrient — way more than you'd ever naturally eat. If your male partner frequently binges on Brazil nuts then maybe get him to lay off, but otherwise, don't choose an antioxidant formula with selenium in it.

SUPPLEMENTS TO SUPPORT MALE FERTILITY

I will preface this section with two reminders: your male partner needs a practitioner, and none of these supplements has been looked at specifically for miscarriage. I cannot tell you the number of times a female who is launching into a major health and wellness plan for her fertility casually asks if her male partner "should take anything for his sperm". We are missing the point here ladies. Supplements don't fix things, and if you are doing a total health and wellness plan to conceive and carry to term, then maybe so should he. Here is a list of supplements to discuss with your male partner's practitioner. Most of them have side-benefits and very few side effects, so choosing the right combination should depend on what extra benefits you are hoping to have.

DHA is one of the two omega-3 fatty acids found in fish. We have seen in the diet research that increasing fish intake improves male fertility, and as it appears, supplementing DHA alone (in higher doses than you'd achieve through diet) improves DNA fragmentation and sperm health in men with infertility[155]. This change takes at least three months of supplementation, so ideally fish oil supplements are part of a longer-term preconception plan.

Maca is a herb that has been studied multiple times for its effect on semen quality and quantity. In both fertile and infertile men, Maca appears to improve markers of better fertility[156]. Tribulus is a plant that has traditionally been used to improve libido in both males and females. In one study, they show improvement not only in sperm parameters but in lean body mass and fat mass of the men who supplemented before their IVF cycle[157]. Win-win perhaps?

Withania is an herb that has been shown to improve stress pathways and increase testosterone[158]. It has shown some promise for male fertility, especially when stress has been implicated as a contributing factor to lower sperm counts.

Vitamin C has always been one of the best-studied antioxidants, even though it is not the strongest antioxidant out there. Most of the research points towards supplemental vitamin C having an impact, even at a low dose. This likely speaks to the little fruit and vegetable intake in most study populations, but it is a cheap and easy supplement. In one of the more specific studies, they used Vitamin C in men who had surgery for varicocele and found that the sperm motility and quality were better in the men who supplemented before and after undergoing the knife than men who took a placebo[151]. 250 mg twice per day is likely all that is needed.

Co-Q10 has been studied more than most antioxidants for sperm quality, and a large review of many studies discourages its use[159]. Why? Because every study has looked at surrogate outcomes (semen) not clinical outcomes (births). It does not mean that it does not work, but it means that we haven't studied it well enough to say without a doubt that it helps to have more babies.

Other antioxidants have been looked at in small or single trials. Be on the lookout for nutrients such as carnitine, probiotics, alpha-lipoic acid, turmeric and resveratrol coming on the scene as important inclusions in a compressive treatment plan for male infertility. As of this moment, I would likely only use them if we had some side-benefits we were after, or if oxidative stress seemed high, or to be a significant contributor to a particular case.

GENERAL HEALTH HABITS

Stress and lack of sleep have both been shown to reduce semen quality[160]. Cortisol directly affects testosterone production, and men who have a shorter sleep duration have higher levels of anti-sperm antibody, which lowers motility and sperm survival. Managing the stress response could be as simple as focusing on self-care, meditation, exercise and good sleep hygiene. If these simple strategies don't work, or if general health needs more of a tune-up, then have your male partner talk to a practitioner (which really, if we haven't got him into an office by this point in the chapter I'm not convincing enough!)

Lastly, advanced paternal age is a significant predictor for miscarriage. One trial looked at 83 couples and found that in couples with a male partner over 40 years of age, 60% of the initially successful IVF cycles ended in miscarriage, whereas only 40% of the cycles with younger dads experienced a miscarriage[161]. Both had very high numbers, but the impact of age was significant.

Food for thought, and if you have an older male partner, then you perhaps want to consider more antioxidant support or aggressive strategies, knowing that age is working against your case.

REFERENCES

1. Ford, H. B. & Schust, D. J. Recurrent Pregnancy Loss: Etiology, Diagnosis, and Therapy. *Rev Obstet Gynecol* **2,** 76–83 (2009).

2. Jaslow, C. R., Carney, J. L. & Kutteh, W. H. Diagnostic factors identified in 1020 women with two versus three or more recurrent pregnancy losses. *Fertil. Steril.* **93,** 1234–1243 (2010).

3. Weghofer, A., Munne, S., Chen, S., Barad, D. & Gleicher, N. Lack of association between polycystic ovary syndrome and embryonic aneuploidy. *Fertil. Steril.* **88,** 900–905 (2007).

4. Luo, L. *et al.* Early miscarriage rate in lean polycystic ovary syndrome women after euploid embryo transfer—a matched-pair study. *Reprod. Biomed. Online* **35,** 576–582 (2017).

5. Palomba, S. *et al.* Decidual Endovascular Trophoblast Invasion in Women with Polycystic Ovary Syndrome: An Experimental Case-Control Study. *J Clin Endocrinol Metab* **97,** 2441–2449 (2012).

6. Cui, N. *et al.* Impact of Body Mass Index on Outcomes of In Vitro Fertilization/Intracytoplasmic Sperm Injection Among Polycystic Ovarian Syndrome Patients. *Cell. Physiol. Biochem.* **39,** 1723–1734 (2016).

7. Mesen, T. B. & Young, S. L. Progesterone and the Luteal Phase. *Obstet Gynecol Clin North Am* **42,** 135–151 (2015).

8. Subrat, P., Santa, S. A. & Vandana, J. The Concepts and Consequences of Early Ovarian Ageing: A Caveat to Women's Health. *J Reprod Infertil* **14,** 3–7 (2013).

9. Green, D. M. *et al.* Ovarian failure and reproductive outcomes after childhood cancer treatment: results from the Childhood Cancer Survivor Study. *J. Clin. Oncol.* **27,** 2374–2381 (2009).

10. Chuang, C. C. *et al.* Age is a better predictor of pregnancy potential than basal follicle-stimulating hormone levels in women undergoing in vitro fertilization. *Fertil. Steril.* **79,** 63–68 (2003).

11. Yuan, X., Lin, H. Y., Wang, Q. & Li, T. C. Is premature ovarian ageing a cause of unexplained recurrent miscarriage? *J Obstet Gynaecol* **32,** 464–466 (2012).

12. Abdalla, H. & Thum, M. Y. An elevated basal FSH reflects a quantitative rather than qualitative decline of the ovarian reserve. *Hum. Reprod.* **19,** 893–898 (2004).

13. Hewlett, M. & Mahalingaiah, S. Update on Primary Ovarian Insufficiency. *Current opinion in endocrinology, diabetes, and obesity* **22,** 483 (2015).

14. Stagnaro-Green, A. *et al.* Guidelines of the American Thyroid Association for the Diagnosis and Management of Thyroid Disease During Pregnancy and Postpartum. *Thyroid* **21,** 1081–1125 (2011).

15. Horacek, J. *et al.* Universal screening detects two-times more thyroid disorders in early pregnancy than targeted high-risk case finding. *Eur. J. Endocrinol.* **163,** 645–650 (2010).

16. Murphy, M. M. Homocysteine: biomarker or cause of adverse pregnancy outcome? *Biomark Med* **1,** 145–157 (2007).

17. Murphy, M. M., Fernandez-Ballart, J. D., Molloy, A. M. & Canals, J. Moderately elevated maternal homocysteine at preconception is inversely associated with cognitive performance in children 4 months and 6 years after birth. *Matern Child Nutr* (2016). doi:10.1111/mcn.12289

18. D'Hooghe, T. M., Debrock, S., Hill, J. A. & Meuleman, C. Endometriosis and subfertility: is the relationship resolved? *Semin. Reprod. Med.* **21,** 243–254 (2003).

19. Hirsch, M. *et al.* Diagnostic accuracy of cancer antigen 125 for endometriosis: a systematic review and meta-analysis. *BJOG* **123,** 1761–1768 (2016).

20. Lathi, R. B. *et al.* The role of serum testosterone in early pregnancy outcome: a comparison in women with and without polycystic ovary syndrome. *J Obstet Gynaecol Can* **36,** 811–816 (2014).

21. Lin, X. F. *et al.* Exploring the significance of sex hormone-binding globulin examination in the treament of women with polycystic ovarian syndrome (PCOS). *Clin Exp Obstet Gynecol* **42,** 315–320 (2015).

22. Pal, L. *et al.* Vitamin D Status Relates to Reproductive Outcome in Women With Polycystic Ovary Syndrome: Secondary Analysis of a Multicenter Randomized Controlled Trial. *J. Clin. Endocrinol. Metab.* **101,** 3027–3035 (2016).

23. Nisenblat, V. *et al.* Blood biomarkers for the non-invasive diagnosis of endometriosis. *Cochrane Database Syst Rev* CD012179 (2016). doi:10.1002/14651858.CD012179

24. Ruan, Y.-Q., Liang, W.-G. & Huang, S.-H. Analysis of laparoscopy on endometriosis patients with high expression of CA125. *Eur Rev Med Pharmacol Sci* **19,** 1334–1337 (2015).

25. Nepomnaschy, P. A. *et al.* Cortisol levels and very early pregnancy loss in humans. *Proc Natl Acad Sci U S A* **103,** 3938–3942 (2006).

26. Jeve, Y. B. & Davies, W. Evidence-based management of recurrent miscarriages. *J Hum Reprod Sci* **7,** 159–169 (2014).

27. Palomba, S. *et al.* Decidual endovascular trophoblast invasion in women with polycystic ovary syndrome: an

experimental case-control study. *J. Clin. Endocrinol. Metab.* **97,** 2441–2449 (2012).

28. Marsh, K. A., Steinbeck, K. S., Atkinson, F. S., Petocz, P. & Brand-Miller, J. C. Effect of a low glycemic index compared with a conventional healthy diet on polycystic ovary syndrome. *Am J Clin Nutr* **92,** 83–92 (2010).

29. An, Y. *et al.* The use of berberine for women with polycystic ovary syndrome undergoing IVF treatment. *Clin. Endocrinol. (Oxf)* **80,** 425–431 (2014).

30. Asadi, M. *et al.* Vitamin D improves endometrial thickness in PCOS women who need intrauterine insemination: a randomized double-blind placebo-controlled trial. *Arch Gynecol Obstet* **289,** 865–870 (2014).

31. Köşüş, A., Köşüş, N., Haktankaçmaz, S. A., Ak, D. & Turhan, N. Ö. Effect of dose and duration of micronized progesterone treatment during the first trimester on incidence of glucose intolerance and on birth weight. *Fetal. Diagn. Ther.* **31,** 49–54 (2012).

32. Moran, L. J. *et al.* Dietary composition in restoring reproductive and metabolic physiology in overweight women with polycystic ovary syndrome. *J. Clin. Endocrinol. Metab.* **88,** 812–819 (2003).

33. Gower, B. A. *et al.* Favourable metabolic effects of a eucaloric lower-carbohydrate diet in women with PCOS. *Clin Endocrinol (Oxf)* **79,** 550–557 (2013).

34. Glueck, C. J. *et al.* Effects of metformin-diet intervention before and throughout pregnancy on obstetric and neonatal outcomes in patients with polycystic ovary syndrome. *Curr Med Res Opin* **29,** 55–62 (2013).

35. Unfer, V., Nestler, J. E., Kamenov, Z. A., Prapas, N. & Facchinetti, F. Effects of Inositol(s) in Women with PCOS: A Systematic Review of Randomized Controlled

Trials. *International Journal of Endocrinology* (2016). doi:10.1155/2016/1849162

36. Salehpour, S. *et al.* A Potential Therapeutic Role of Myoinositol in the Metabolic and Cardiovascular Profile of PCOS Iranian Women Aged between 30 and 40 Years. *Int J Endocrinol* **2016,** 7493147 (2016).

37. Farren, M. *et al.* The Prevention of Gestational Diabetes Mellitus With Antenatal Oral Inositol Supplementation: A Randomized Controlled Trial. *Diabetes Care* **40,** 759–763 (2017).

38. Glueck, C. J., Streicher, P. & Wang, P. Treatment of polycystic ovary syndrome with insulin-lowering agents. *Expert Opin Pharmacother* **3,** 1177–1189 (2002).

39. Al-Biate, M. A. S. Effect of metformin on early pregnancy loss in women with polycystic ovary syndrome. *Taiwan J Obstet Gynecol* **54,** 266–269 (2015).

40. Practice Committee of the American Society for Reproductive Medicine. The clinical relevance of luteal phase deficiency: a committee opinion. *Fertil. Steril.* **98,** 1112–1117 (2012).

41. Halbreich, U. The diagnosis of premenstrual syndromes and premenstrual dysphoric disorder--clinical procedures and research perspectives. *Gynecol. Endocrinol.* **19,** 320–334 (2004).

42. Milewicz, A. *et al.* [Vitex agnus castus extract in the treatment of luteal phase defects due to latent hyperprolactinemia. Results of a randomized placebo-controlled double-blind study]. *Arzneimittelforschung* **43,** 752–756 (1993).

43. Henmi, H. *et al.* Effects of ascorbic acid supplementation on serum progesterone levels in patients with a luteal phase defect. *Fertil. Steril.* **80,** 459–461 (2003).

44. Taketani, T. *et al.* Protective role of melatonin in progesterone production by human luteal cells. *J. Pineal Res.* **51,** 207–213 (2011).

45. Tamura, H. *et al.* Melatonin as a free radical scavenger in the ovarian follicle. *Endocr. J.* **60,** 1–13 (2013).

46. Eryilmaz, O. G. *et al.* Melatonin improves the oocyte and the embryo in IVF patients with sleep disturbances, but does not improve the sleeping problems. *J. Assist. Reprod. Genet.* **28,** 815–820 (2011).

47. Nishihara, T. *et al.* Oral melatonin supplementation improves oocyte and embryo quality in women undergoing in vitro fertilization-embryo transfer. *Gynecol. Endocrinol.* **30,** 359–362 (2014).

48. Weisz, G. & Knaapen, L. Diagnosing and treating premenstrual syndrome in five western nations. *Soc Sci Med* **68,** 1498–1505 (2009).

49. Check, J. H. Luteal phase support for in vitro fertilization-embryo transfer--present and future methods to improve successful implantation. *Clin Exp Obstet Gynecol* **39,** 422–428 (2012).

50. Ismail, A. M., Abbas, A. M., Ali, M. K. & Amin, A. F. Peri-conceptional progesterone treatment in women with unexplained recurrent miscarriage: a randomized double-blind placebo-controlled trial. *J. Matern. Fetal. Neonatal. Med.* 1–7 (2017). doi:10.1080/14767058.2017.1286315

51. Chen, H., Fu, J. & Huang, W. Dopamine agonists for preventing future miscarriage in women with idiopathic hyperprolactinemia and recurrent miscarriage history. *Cochrane Database Syst Rev* **7,** CD008883 (2016).

52. Fadhlaoui, A., Bouquet de la Jolinière, J. & Feki, A. Endometriosis and Infertility: How and When to Treat? *Front Surg* **1,** (2014).

53. Dunselman, G. a. J. *et al.* ESHRE guideline: management of women with endometriosis. *Hum. Reprod.* **29,** 400–412 (2014).
54. Santanam, N., Kavtaradze, N., Murphy, A., Dominguez, C. & Parthasarathy, S. Antioxidant Supplementation Reduces Endometriosis Related Pelvic Pain in Humans. *Transl Res* **161,** 189–195 (2013).
55. Schwertner, A. *et al.* Efficacy of melatonin in the treatment of endometriosis: a phase II, randomized, double-blind, placebo-controlled trial. *Pain* **154,** 874–881 (2013).
56. Khanaki, K. *et al.* Evaluation of the relationship between endometriosis and omega-3 and omega-6 polyunsaturated fatty acids. *Iran. Biomed. J.* **16,** 38–43 (2012).
57. Miyashita, M. *et al.* Effects of 1,25-dihydroxy vitamin D3 on endometriosis. *J. Clin. Endocrinol. Metab.* jc20161515 (2016). doi:10.1210/jc.2016-1515
58. Sayegh, L., Fuleihan, G. E.-H. & Nassar, A. H. Vitamin D in endometriosis: a causative or confounding factor? *Metab. Clin. Exp.* **63,** 32–41 (2014).
59. Erten, O. U. *et al.* Vitamin C is effective for the prevention and regression of endometriotic implants in an experimentally induced rat model of endometriosis. *Taiwan J Obstet Gynecol* **55,** 251–257 (2016).
60. Rier, S. & Foster, W. G. Environmental dioxins and endometriosis. *Toxicol. Sci.* **70,** 161–170 (2002).
61. Bruner-Tran, K. L. & Osteen, K. G. Dioxin-like PCBs and Endometriosis. *Syst Biol Reprod Med* **56,** 132–146 (2010).
62. Mier-Cabrera, J. *et al.* Women with endometriosis improved their peripheral antioxidant markers after the application of a high antioxidant diet. *Reproductive Biology and Endocrinology* **7,** 54 (2009).

63. Parazzini, F. *et al.* Selected food intake and risk of endometriosis. *Hum. Reprod.* **19,** 1755–1759 (2004).
64. Missmer, S. A. *et al.* A prospective study of dietary fat consumption and endometriosis risk. *Hum. Reprod.* **25,** 1528–1535 (2010).
65. Tsuchiya, M. *et al.* Effect of soy isoflavones on endometriosis: interaction with estrogen receptor 2 gene polymorphism. *Epidemiology* **18,** 402–408 (2007).
66. Nagata, C., Takatsuka, N., Kawakami, N. & Shimizu, H. Soy product intake and premenopausal hysterectomy in a follow-up study of Japanese women. *Eur J Clin Nutr* **55,** 773–777 (2001).
67. Upson, K., Sathyanarayana, S., Scholes, D. & Holt, V. L. Early-life factors and endometriosis risk. *Fertil. Steril.* **104,** 964-971.e5 (2015).
68. Matorras, R., Elorriaga, M. A., Pijoan, J. I., Ramón, O. & Rodríguez-Escudero, F. J. Recurrence of endometriosis in women with bilateral adnexectomy (with or without total hysterectomy) who received hormone replacement therapy. *Fertil. Steril.* **77,** 303–308 (2002).
69. Chen, J. *et al.* Efficacy and safety of remifemin on perimenopausal symptoms induced by post-operative GnRH-a therapy for endometriosis: a randomized study versus tibolone. *Med. Sci. Monit.* **20,** 1950–1957 (2014).
70. Wei, M., Cheng, Y., Bu, H., Zhao, Y. & Zhao, W. Length of Menstrual Cycle and Risk of Endometriosis: A Meta-Analysis of 11 Case-Control Studies. *Medicine (Baltimore)* **95,** e2922 (2016).
71. Singh, A. K., Chattopadhyay, R., Chakravarty, B. & Chaudhury, K. Altered circulating levels of matrix metalloproteinases 2 and 9 and their inhibitors and effect of progesterone supplementation in women with

endometriosis undergoing in vitro fertilization. *Fertil. Steril.* **100,** 127-134.e1 (2013).

72. Chakraborty, P. *et al.* Recurrent pregnancy loss in polycystic ovary syndrome: role of hyperhomocysteinemia and insulin resistance. *PLoS ONE* **8,** e64446 (2013).

73. Ayar, A., Celik, H., Ozcelik, O. & Kelestimur, H. Homocysteine-induced enhancement of spontaneous contractions of myometrium isolated from pregnant women. *Acta Obstet Gynecol Scand* **82,** 789–793 (2003).

74. de la Calle, M. *et al.* Homocysteine, folic acid and B-group vitamins in obstetrics and gynaecology. *Eur. J. Obstet. Gynecol. Reprod. Biol.* **107,** 125–134 (2003).

75. Boas, W. V., Gonçalves, R. O., Costa, O. L. N. & Goncalves, M. S. Metabolism and gene polymorphisms of the folate pathway in Brazilian women with history of recurrent abortion. *Rev Bras Ginecol Obstet* **37,** 71–76 (2015).

76. Willems, F. F., Boers, G. H. J., Blom, H. J., Aengevaeren, W. R. M. & Verheugt, F. W. A. Pharmacokinetic study on the utilisation of 5-methyltetrahydrofolate and folic acid in patients with coronary artery disease. *Br. J. Pharmacol.* **141,** 825–830 (2004).

77. Venn, B. J., Green, T. J., Moser, R. & Mann, J. I. Comparison of the effect of low-dose supplementation with L-5-methyltetrahydrofolate or folic acid on plasma homocysteine: a randomized placebo-controlled study. *Am. J. Clin. Nutr.* **77,** 658–662 (2003).

78. Atkinson, W., Elmslie, J., Lever, M., Chambers, S. T. & George, P. M. Dietary and supplementary betaine: acute effects on plasma betaine and homocysteine concentrations under standard and postmethionine load conditions in healthy male subjects. *Am J Clin Nutr* **87,** 577–585 (2008).

79. Brouwer, I. A., Verhoef, P. & Urgert, R. Betaine Supplementation and Plasma Homocysteine in Healthy Volunteers. *Arch Intern Med* **160**, 2546–2546 (2000).

80. Wallace, J. M. W. *et al.* Choline supplementation and measures of choline and betaine status: a randomised, controlled trial in postmenopausal women. *Br. J. Nutr.* **108**, 1264–1271 (2012).

81. Debiève, F. *et al.* To treat or not to treat euthyroid autoimmune disorder during pregnancy? *Gynecol. Obstet. Invest.* **67**, 178–182 (2009).

82. Vissenberg, R. *et al.* Effect of levothyroxine on live birth rate in euthyroid women with recurrent miscarriage and TPO antibodies (T4-LIFE study). *Contemp Clin Trials* (2015). doi:10.1016/j.cct.2015.08.005

83. Pradhan, M., Anand, B., Singh, N. & Mehrotra, M. Thyroid peroxidase antibody in hypothyroidism: it's effect on pregnancy. *J. Matern. Fetal. Neonatal. Med.* **26**, 581–583 (2013).

84. Bhattacharyya, R. *et al.* Anti-thyroid peroxidase antibody positivity during early pregnancy is associated with pregnancy complications and maternal morbidity in later life. *J Nat Sci Biol Med* **6**, 402–405 (2015).

85. Mazokopakis, E. E. *et al.* Effects of 12 months treatment with L-selenomethionine on serum anti-TPO Levels in Patients with Hashimoto's thyroiditis. *Thyroid* **17**, 609–612 (2007).

86. Wichman, J., Winther, K. H., Bonnema, S. J. & Hegedüs, L. Selenium Supplementation Significantly Reduces Thyroid Autoantibody Levels in Patients with Chronic Autoimmune Thyroiditis: A Systematic Review and Meta-Analysis. *Thyroid* **26**, 1681–1692 (2016).

87. Chaudhary, S. *et al.* Vitamin D supplementation reduces thyroid peroxidase antibody levels in patients with

autoimmune thyroid disease: An open-labeled randomized controlled trial. *Indian J Endocrinol Metab* **20,** 391–398 (2016).

88. Liontiris, M. I. & Mazokopakis, E. E. A concise review of Hashimoto thyroiditis (HT) and the importance of iodine, selenium, vitamin D and gluten on the autoimmunity and dietary management of HT patients.Points that need more investigation. *Hell J Nucl Med* **20,** 51–56 (2017).

89. Hoang, T. D., Olsen, C. H., Mai, V. Q., Clyde, P. W. & Shakir, M. K. M. Desiccated thyroid extract compared with levothyroxine in the treatment of hypothyroidism: a randomized, double-blind, crossover study. *J. Clin. Endocrinol. Metab.* **98,** 1982–1990 (2013).

90. Seshadri, S. & Sunkara, S. K. Natural killer cells in female infertility and recurrent miscarriage: a systematic review and meta-analysis. *Hum. Reprod. Update* **20,** 429–438 (2014).

91. Moffett, A., Regan, L. & Braude, P. Natural killer cells, miscarriage, and infertility. *BMJ* **329,** 1283–1285 (2004).

92. Carta, G., Iovenitti, P. & Falciglia, K. Recurrent miscarriage associated with antiphospholipid antibodies: prophylactic treatment with low-dose aspirin and fish oil derivates. *Clin Exp Obstet Gynecol* **32,** 49–51 (2005).

93. Domar, A. D., Conboy, L., Denardo-Roney, J. & Rooney, K. L. Lifestyle behaviors in women undergoing in vitro fertilization: a prospective study. *Fertil. Steril.* **97,** 697-701.e1 (2012).

94. Domar, A. D., Rooney, K. L., Milstein, M. & Conboy, L. Lifestyle habits of 12,800 IVF patients: Prevalence of negative lifestyle behaviors, and impact of region and insurance coverage. *Hum Fertil (Camb)* **18,** 253–257 (2015).

95. Klonoff-Cohen, H., Lam-Kruglick, P. & Gonzalez, C. Effects of maternal and paternal alcohol consumption

on the success rates of in vitro fertilization and gamete intrafallopian transfer. *Fertil. Steril.* **79,** 330–339 (2003).

96. Stefanidou, E. M., Caramellino, L., Patriarca, A. & Menato, G. Maternal caffeine consumption and sine causa recurrent miscarriage. *Eur. J. Obstet. Gynecol. Reprod. Biol.* **158,** 220–224 (2011).

97. Cnattingius, S. *et al.* Caffeine intake and the risk of first-trimester spontaneous abortion. *N. Engl. J. Med.* **343,** 1839–1845 (2000).

98. Chavarro, J. E., Rich-Edwards, J. W., Rosner, B. A. & Willett, W. C. Protein intake and ovulatory infertility. *Am. J. Obstet. Gynecol.* **198,** 210.e1–7 (2008).

99. Chavarro, J. E., Rich-Edwards, J. W., Rosner, B. A. & Willett, W. C. Iron intake and risk of ovulatory infertility. *Obstet Gynecol* **108,** 1145–1152 (2006).

100. Chavarro, J. E., Rich-Edwards, J. W., Rosner, B. & Willett, W. C. A prospective study of dairy foods intake and anovulatory infertility. *Hum. Reprod.* **22,** 1340–1347 (2007).

101. Chavarro, J. E., Rich-Edwards, J. W., Rosner, B. A. & Willett, W. C. Dietary fatty acid intakes and the risk of ovulatory infertility. *Am. J. Clin. Nutr.* **85,** 231–237 (2007).

102. Vujkovic, M. *et al.* The preconception Mediterranean dietary pattern in couples undergoing in vitro fertilization/intracytoplasmic sperm injection treatment increases the chance of pregnancy. *Fertil. Steril.* **94,** 2096–2101 (2010).

103. Chavarro, J. E., Rich-Edwards, J. W., Rosner, B. A. & Willett, W. C. A prospective study of dietary carbohydrate quantity and quality in relation to risk of ovulatory infertility. *Eur J Clin Nutr* **63,** 78–86 (2009).

104. Bø, K. *et al.* Exercise and pregnancy in recreational and elite athletes: 2016 evidence summary from the IOC expert group meeting, Lausanne. Part 2-the effect of exercise

on the fetus, labour and birth. *Br J Sports Med* (2016). doi:10.1136/bjsports-2016-096810

105. Ammon Avalos, L., Kaskutas, L. A., Block, G. & Li, D.-K. Do multivitamin supplements modify the relationship between prenatal alcohol intake and miscarriage? *Am. J. Obstet. Gynecol.* **201,** 563.e1–9 (2009).

106. Andreoli, L. *et al.* Vitamin D and antiphospholipid syndrome. *Lupus* **21,** 736–740 (2012).

107. Balogun, O. O. *et al.* Vitamin supplementation for preventing miscarriage. *Cochrane Database Syst Rev* CD004073 (2016). doi:10.1002/14651858.CD004073.pub4

108. Piantoni, S., Andreoli, L., Allegri, F., Meroni, P. L. & Tincani, A. Low levels of vitamin D are common in primary antiphospholipid syndrome with thrombotic disease. *Reumatismo* **64,** 307–313 (2012).

109. Bärebring, L. *et al.* Trajectory of vitamin D status during pregnancy in relation to neonatal birth size and fetal survival: a prospective cohort study. *BMC Pregnancy Childbirth* **18,** 51 (2018).

110. Grzechocinska, B., Dabrowski, F. A., Cyganek, A. & Wielgos, M. The role of vitamin D in impaired fertility treatment. *Neuro Endocrinol. Lett.* **34,** 756–762 (2013).

111. Wang, L.-Q. *et al.* Women with Recurrent Miscarriage Have Decreased Expression of 25-Hydroxyvitamin D3-1α-Hydroxylase by the Fetal-Maternal Interface. *PLoS ONE* **11,** e0165589 (2016).

112. Mazokopakis, E. E. *et al.* Is vitamin D related to pathogenesis and treatment of Hashimoto's thyroiditis? *Hell J Nucl Med* **18,** 222–227 (2015).

113. Mier-Cabrera, J. *et al.* Effect of vitamins C and E supplementation on peripheral oxidative stress markers and pregnancy rate in women with endometriosis. *Int J Gynaecol Obstet* **100,** 252–256 (2008).

114. Mohebbi, M., Akbari, S. A. A., Mahmodi, Z. & Nasiri, M. Comparison between the lifestyles of university students with and without premenstrual syndromes. *Electron Physician* **9,** 4489–4496 (2017).
115. Gernand, A. D., Schulze, K. J., Stewart, C. P., West, K. P. & Christian, P. Micronutrient deficiencies in pregnancy worldwide: health effects and prevention. *Nat Rev Endocrinol* **12,** 274–289 (2016).
116. Feodor Nilsson, S., Andersen, P. K., Strandberg-Larsen, K. & Nybo Andersen, A.-M. Risk factors for miscarriage from a prevention perspective: a nationwide follow-up study. *BJOG* **121,** 1375–1384 (2014).
117. Lawson, C. C. et al. Rotating shift work and menstrual cycle characteristics. *Epidemiology* **22,** 305–312 (2011).
118. Kim, M. K. et al. Does supplementation of in-vitro culture medium with melatonin improve IVF outcome in PCOS? *Reprod. Biomed. Online* **26,** 22–29 (2013).
119. Fernando, S. & Rombauts, L. Melatonin: shedding light on infertility?—a review of the recent literature. *J Ovarian Res* **7,** (2014).
120. Taketani, T. et al. Protective role of melatonin in progesterone production by human luteal cells. *J. Pineal Res.* **51,** 207–213 (2011).
121. Li, Y., Liu, H., Sun, J., Tian, Y. & Li, C. Effect of melatonin on the peripheral T lymphocyte cell cycle and levels of reactive oxygen species in patients with premature ovarian failure. *Exp Ther Med* **12,** 3589–3594 (2016).
122. Pacchiarotti, A., Gianfranco Carlomagno, Antonini, G. & Pacchiarotti, A. Effect of myo-inositol and melatonin versus myo-inositol, in a randomized controlled trial, for improving in vitro fertilization of patients with polycystic ovarian syndrome. *Gynecol. Endocrinol.* **32,** 69–73 (2016).

123. Moran, L. J., Tsagareli, V., Noakes, M. & Norman, R. Altered Preconception Fatty Acid Intake Is Associated with Improved Pregnancy Rates in Overweight and Obese Women Undertaking in Vitro Fertilisation. *Nutrients* **8**, (2016).
124. Hammiche, F. *et al.* Tailored preconceptional dietary and lifestyle counselling in a tertiary outpatient clinic in The Netherlands. *Hum. Reprod.* **26**, 2432–2441 (2011).
125. Lazzarin, N. *et al.* Low-dose aspirin and omega-3 fatty acids improve uterine artery blood flow velocity in women with recurrent miscarriage due to impaired uterine perfusion. *Fertil. Steril.* **92**, 296–300 (2009).
126. Pirola, I., Gandossi, E., Agosti, B., Delbarba, A. & Cappelli, C. Selenium supplementation could restore euthyroidism in subclinical hypothyroid patients with autoimmune thyroiditis. *Endokrynol Pol* **67**, 567–571 (2016).
127. van Zuuren, E. J., Albusta, A. Y., Fedorowicz, Z., Carter, B. & Pijl, H. Selenium supplementation for Hashimoto's thyroiditis. *Cochrane Database Syst Rev* CD010223 (2013). doi:10.1002/14651858.CD010223.pub2
128. Andrews, M. A. *et al.* Dietary factors and luteal phase deficiency in healthy eumenorrheic women. *Hum Reprod* **30**, 1942–1951 (2015).
129. Jamilian, M. *et al.* Metabolic response to selenium supplementation in women with polycystic ovary syndrome: a randomized, double-blind, placebo-controlled trial. *Clin. Endocrinol. (Oxf)* **82**, 885–891 (2015).
130. Mohammad Hosseinzadeh, F., Hosseinzadeh-Attar, M. J., Yekaninejad, M. S. & Rashidi, B. Effects of selenium supplementation on glucose homeostasis and free androgen index in women with polycystic ovary syndrome:

A randomized, double blinded, placebo controlled clinical trial. *J Trace Elem Med Biol* **34,** 56–61 (2016).

131. Thakker, D., Raval, A., Patel, I. & Walia, R. N-Acetylcysteine for Polycystic Ovary Syndrome: A Systematic Review and Meta-Analysis of Randomized Controlled Clinical Trials. *Obstet Gynecol Int* **2015,** (2015).

132. Nasr, A. Effect of N-acetyl-cysteine after ovarian drilling in clomiphene citrate-resistant PCOS women: a pilot study. *Reprod. Biomed. Online* **20,** 403–409 (2010).

133. McDonald, S. D., Perkins, S. L., Jodouin, C. A. & Walker, M. C. Folate levels in pregnant women who smoke: an important gene/environment interaction. *Am. J. Obstet. Gynecol.* **187,** 620–625 (2002).

134. Hübner, U. *et al.* Low serum vitamin B12 is associated with recurrent pregnancy loss in Syrian women. *Clin. Chem. Lab. Med.* **46,** 1265–1269 (2008).

135. Xu, Q. *et al.* Sex Hormone Metabolism and Threatened Abortion. *Med Sci Monit* **23,** 5041–5048 (2017).

136. Mamas, L. & Mamas, E. Dehydroepiandrosterone supplementation in assisted reproduction: rationale and results. *Curr. Opin. Obstet. Gynecol.* **21,** 306–308 (2009).

137. Mesen, T. B. & Young, S. L. Progesterone and the Luteal Phase. *Obstet Gynecol Clin North Am* **42,** 135–151 (2015).

138. Hefler, L., Grimm, C., Tempfer, C. & Reinthaller, A. Treatment with vaginal progesterone in women with low-grade cervical dysplasia: a phase II trial. *Anticancer Res.* **30,** 1257–1261 (2010).

139. Ding, J. *et al.* FDA-approved medications that impair human spermatogenesis. *Oncotarget* **8,** 10714–10725 (2016).

140. Drobnis, E. Z. & Nangia, A. K. Psychotropics and Male Reproduction. *Adv. Exp. Med. Biol.* **1034,** 63–101 (2017).

REFERENCES

141. Huijgen, N. A. *et al.* Effect of Medications for Gastric Acid-Related Symptoms on Total Motile Sperm Count and Concentration: A Case-Control Study in Men of Subfertile Couples from the Netherlands. *Drug Saf* **40,** 241–248 (2017).

142. Drobnis, E. Z. & Nangia, A. K. Pain Medications and Male Reproduction. *Adv. Exp. Med. Biol.* **1034,** 39–57 (2017).

143. Wu, F. C. W. *et al.* Hypothalamic-pituitary-testicular axis disruptions in older men are differentially linked to age and modifiable risk factors: the European Male Aging Study. *J. Clin. Endocrinol. Metab.* **93,** 2737–2745 (2008).

144. Oliveira, P. F., Sousa, M., Silva, B. M., Monteiro, M. P. & Alves, M. G. Obesity, energy balance and spermatogenesis. *Reproduction* (2017). doi:10.1530/REP-17-0018

145. Strain, G. W. *et al.* Effect of massive weight loss on hypothalamic-pituitary-gonadal function in obese men. *J. Clin. Endocrinol. Metab.* **66,** 1019–1023 (1988).

146. Salas-Huetos, A., Bulló, M. & Salas-Salvadó, J. Dietary patterns, foods and nutrients in male fertility parameters and fecundability: a systematic review of observational studies. *Hum. Reprod. Update* **23,** 371–389 (2017).

147. Yamamoto, Y. *et al.* The effects of tomato juice on male infertility. *Asia Pac J Clin Nutr* **26,** 65–71 (2017).

148. Mehdipour, M., Daghigh Kia, H., Najafi, A., Vaseghi Dodaran, H. & García-Álvarez, O. Effect of green tea (Camellia sinensis) extract and pre-freezing equilibration time on the post-thawing quality of ram semen cryopreserved in a soybean lecithin-based extender. *Cryobiology* **73,** 297–303 (2016).

149. Fedder, M. D. K. *et al.* An extract of pomegranate fruit and galangal rhizome increases the numbers of motile

sperm: a prospective, randomised, controlled, double-blinded trial. *PLoS ONE* **9,** e108532 (2014).

150. Aldemir, M., Okulu, E., Neşelioğlu, S., Erel, O. & Kayıgil, O. Pistachio diet improves erectile function parameters and serum lipid profiles in patients with erectile dysfunction. *Int. J. Impot. Res.* **23,** 32–38 (2011).

151. Akmal, M. *et al.* Improvement in human semen quality after oral supplementation of vitamin C. *J Med Food* **9,** 440–442 (2006).

152. Rafiee, B., Morowvat, M. H. & Rahimi-Ghalati, N. Comparing the Effectiveness of Dietary Vitamin C and Exercise Interventions on Fertility Parameters in Normal Obese Men. *Urol J* **13,** 2635–2639 (2016).

153. Kim, N. *et al.* Effect of lipid metabolism on male fertility. *Biochem. Biophys. Res. Commun.* **485,** 686–692 (2017).

154. Karmon, A. E. *et al.* Male caffeine and alcohol intake in relation to semen parameters and in vitro fertilization outcomes among fertility patients. *Andrology* **5,** 354–361 (2017).

155. Martínez-Soto, J. C. *et al.* Dietary supplementation with docosahexaenoic acid (DHA) improves seminal antioxidant status and decreases sperm DNA fragmentation. *Syst Biol Reprod Med* **62,** 387–395 (2016).

156. Lee, M. S., Lee, H. W., You, S. & Ha, K.-T. The use of maca (Lepidium meyenii) to improve semen quality: A systematic review. *Maturitas* **92,** 64–69 (2016).

157. Salgado, R. M. *et al.* Effect of oral administration of Tribulus terrestris extract on semen quality and body fat index of infertile men. *Andrologia* **49,** (2017).

158. Sengupta, P. *et al.* Role of Withania somnifera (Ashwagandha) in the management of male infertility. *Reprod. Biomed. Online* (2017). doi:10.1016/j.rbmo.2017.11.007

159. Lafuente, R. *et al.* Coenzyme Q10 and male infertility: a meta-analysis. *J Assist Reprod Genet* **30,** 1147–1156 (2013).
160. Liu, M.-M. *et al.* Sleep Deprivation and Late Bedtime Impair Sperm Health Through Increasing Antisperm Antibody Production: A Prospective Study of 981 Healthy Men. *Med. Sci. Monit.* **23,** 1842–1848 (2017).
161. Kaarouch, I. *et al.* Paternal age: Negative impact on sperm genome decays and IVF outcomes after 40 years. *Mol. Reprod. Dev.* **85,** 271–280 (2018).

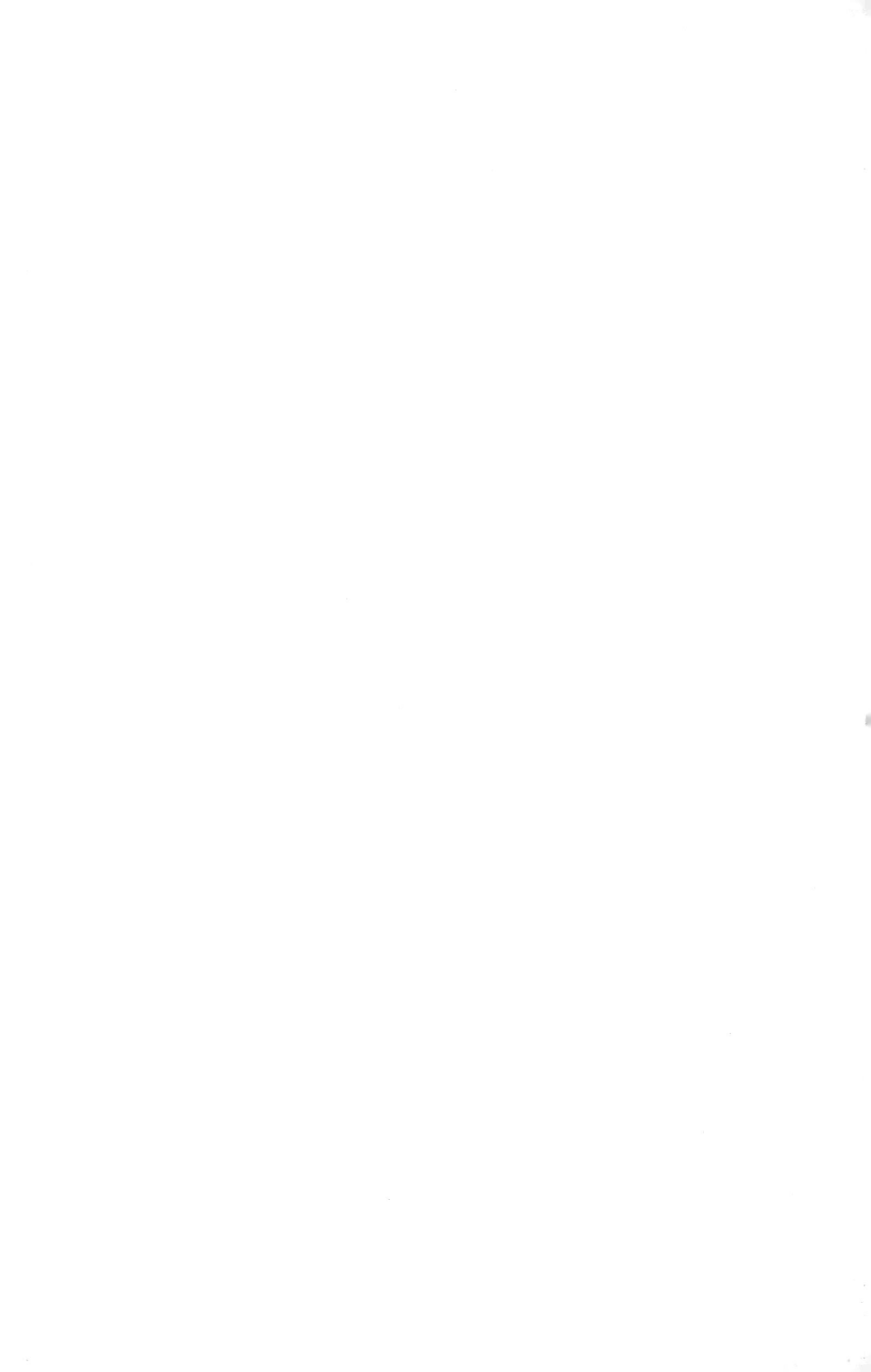

Manufactured by Amazon.ca
Bolton, ON